AUTHOR'S NOTE

It had been several years since the original publication of *Growing Old Is Not for Sissies,* and I found myself thinking a lot about some of these amazingly durable old friends and wondering whatever had happened to them. I remembered how much fun it had been to photograph the burly open-water swimmer Joe Bruno, in his seventies at the time, after he had braved the chilly waters of San Francisco Bay. And I recalled how impressed I had been when I first met Eleanor Hyndman, a short and wiry lady of eighty who practiced karate and wrote lovely poetry. She had been wearing her gi with a purple belt and kicking her coach in the belly while uttering fearful grunts.

So, I decided to take another look and some more pictures to see if the years had slowed them down as much as they had me. My initial telephone calls turned up the inevitable bad news: a few of those iron men and women had died. They had seemed almost immortal to me when I photographed them. But the others I revisited are hale, hearty, and as vigorous as they were the first time around. They continue to thrive on physical challenge, exercise, and the outdoor life. They have survived numerous life crises, some terrible, but somehow retain their enthusiasm and a boundless joie de vivre.

Joe Bruno is eighty-three and still swimming across the treacherous Golden Gate. Eleanor Hyndman is ninety, has advanced to a brown belt in karate, and is still kicking and writing poetry. John Turner, at seventy-nine, displays his sculptured bodybuilder's torso in Nike commercials. And, at age ninety-one, Helen Zechmeister is still wowing the young guys at the gym when she powerlifts more than twice her weight.

My former subjects had all become celebrities after appearing in the first book. Many had appeared on television and radio, and newspaper articles had been written about them. They clearly loved the attention and were ideal subjects for me to shoot again for this second book. In addition, my old friends introduced me to their comrades and competitors. I photographed them, too.

As I got to know my subjects, they told me their stories. They all firmly believe that sports have enhanced their lives—and in some cases have actually cured illnesses and saved sanity. Seventy-six-year-old long-distance runner Fred Ullner was an "overweight, alcoholic, pot-smoking pill popper" when he woke up in the hospital emergency room about ten years ago with a failing liver after a lifetime of hard drinking. The doctors told him he was dying. He took that as a wake-up call, took the pledge, joined Alcoholics Anonymous, and has been running and in good health ever since. Anna Halprin, an exquisitely graceful seventy-five-year-old dancer, is absolutely certain that she beat cancer through the healing powers of dance. Others, like ninety-four-year-old Rose Schwartz, just love the activity. Rose shares it with hundreds of students in the aerobic dance classes she leads five times a week. Ed Longner, ninety-three, stands on his head as a technique for "reverse aging." It seems to work: he is spry as a bird. Besides standing on his head every day, he lifts weights regularly and bowls competitively.

These are extraordinary people, blessed by nature with good genes and possessing an optimistic attitude and the ability to relish the almost impossibly hard work it takes to stay young. During the two years it took to photograph new subjects and reshoot old friends, I was repeatedly struck by how happy these people are. It may be the luck of their good health, the wisdom of age, or a combination of both, but they are obviously and enthusiastically happy. I think it shows in their faces.

—*Etta Clark*

ACKNOWLEDGMENTS

Over the ten years since the first edition of *Growing Old Is Not for Sissies* came out, I have had so much positive reaction that doing a sequel seemed only natural. I want to thank those people who encouraged me to go out and photograph again and my wonderful subjects, who gave me so much of their time and cooperation. Special thanks go to Steve and to my daughters, Nina, Nicki, and Kim, for their love and caring and good advice. Many thanks also to Kevin Leary, my good friend and a journalist, who helped me with my writing, and to his wife, Woody (owner of First Street Books in Kentfield, California), my best friend and enthusiastic supporter; to Linda Connor, my former teacher, who helped me edit my photographs; to Kirk Anspach of Graphics Resources, who did the excellent printing of photographs for this book; to Tom Burke of Pomegranate Artbooks, who took a chance on my idea ten years ago; and to Jill Anderson and Pat Harris, for their editorial assistance.

—*E. C.*

INTRODUCTION

It is a discovery we make at different times of life. It dawns on us that the body is aging but, amazingly, the mind isn't. It stays stubbornly young—in my case, I would say about nineteen. The sober citizen who stares back from my shaving mirror with graven brow conceals the antic youth within, green as a shoot and callow still. It is perplexing. That young man (really no more than a boy) can't understand how he has ended up in the driver's seat of a model with so many miles on it. Hard miles, judging from appearances.

This inner me could easily live as before in that glorious springtime of life. Hard exercise by day, heedless carousal late into the night, yet rising with a glad cry to greet the new day. He never tired, that young barbarian within. What capacity for fun compared with the decrepit impostor the world now witnesses. Soon enough this party will be hobbling with a stick, mouth open to draw in air through unconvincing dentition.

This disjunction between the inner and outer selves—the one evergreen and anchored in time and the other adrift toward inevitable conclusions—is what struck the photographer Etta Clark. Like all artists, she sees with a fresh eye. Hers was the discovery in lovely Marin County, California, where the mania for fitness among young and middle-aged is akin to religious ecstasy, that here and there were older people ("seniors," I suppose we must say) who had simply made up their minds to stand their ground against time's predation. Let skin sag and wrinkle; they would keep the muscles beneath supple by working them as hard as in youth. Or harder: in the past, physical exercise didn't have the cachet it does now. Some of the older women, in fact, were firmly told in girlhood that ladies didn't sweat.

Clark's most famous image, and my favorite, seemed at first like a clever bit of morphing. An ancient's head with snowy Vandyke beard had been arrestingly mounted on the body of a flat-bellied young athlete. An ironic statement, perhaps, about how youth is squandered on the young. But in fact it was an undoctored photograph of John Turner, who was sixty-seven when it was taken. He had the jock's insouciant slouch, head tilted to one side. "So, what do you think?" he seemed to ask. But the eyes told another story. He was satisfied, whatever conflict there was with opinion on how men are supposed to look when they rise from the rocking chair. If you found it (let's say) unconventional, that was your problem. He was a psychiatrist by training and accustomed to listening to problems. Etta photographed Turner again for this book. He is little altered in the decade that has passed.

A T-shirt I recently saw said, "Eat Right. Stay Fit. Die Anyway." Well, yes. None of the recent discoveries in medicine and nutrition alters the hard truth about that third proposition. We have our brief mayfly's glimmer in the material world and then disappear into the mystery. But people are living longer. And there seems no argument that regular exercise keeps lives better longer. The subjects of Clark's photography have taken that small nugget of wisdom to the next level. If some exercise is good, does it not follow that more is better? The elderly athletes in this book (they range in age from fifty-two to one hundred) cleave through straits and bays, run marathons, practice martial arts, dance aerobically or with taps on their shoes. Some gallop horses; others compete in track or swimming meets or pound younger sparring mates with boxing gloves.

Exercise may not be the elixir Ponce de Leon sought, that fabled draught from the Fountain of Youth, but it appears to slow the aging process and may have restorative value. Many of the people in Clark's book are cancer survivors. And who would not be exalted by the example of the remarkable man on the cover, whom Clark discovered in Maui? He has been riding waves on surfboards all his life. When the mood takes him, he paddles out to catch a comber even today, at the age of eighty-three. The awed young surfers respectfully make way for this legendary figure. Reason for awe is not confined to his footwork on big boards: he has a six-year-old son (shown in another photograph). I would not bet against his becoming the first centenarian surfer. In that event, Clark no doubt will photograph him for a revised edition of this book.

The body is a machine with capacities greater than was previously understood, but it is vital to keep the rust off the moving parts. Seemingly, it doesn't matter what you do in the way of exercise, only that you do. California is the starting place of trends that are fated to spread across the rest of the country, and Marin County (Clark's home) is where a good many have begun for California. So it seems a certainty that the senior-as-athlete phenomenon will take root across the land.

One mission of art (there are many) is to inspire. In her photographs, Clark inspires us to realize that whatever our age, it is never too late to rise from our couches, turn off the television, and begin to exercise. All else will follow.

—Jerry Carroll

Look to this day
For it is life
The very life of life.
In its brief course lie
All the realities and verities of existence:
The bliss of growth,
The splendor of action,
The glory of power.
For yesterday is but a dream
And tomorrow is only a vision,
But today, well lived,
Makes every yesterday a dream of happiness
And every tomorrow a vision of hope.
Look well therefore to this day.

—Kalidasa, fourth-century Indian playwright

JOE BRUNO

Rough-water swimmer, age 83

Joe Bruno was the guy who got me started on my first book—ten years ago. A decade older but tough as ever, he still swims in the cold, rough waters of San Francisco Bay every day. He has done the 1.25-mile Golden Gate swim sixty-three times, the first time in 1933.

He added up his races for me: 363 competitive swims, 2,659 competitive miles. The "number one" medal around his neck was given to him by his girlfriend.

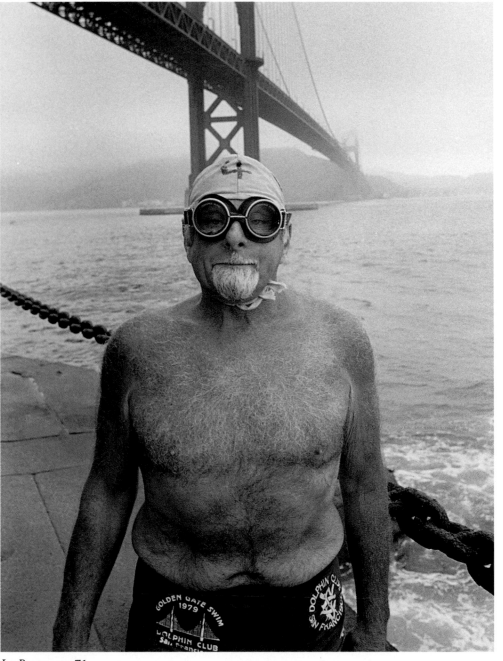

Joe Bruno, age 71

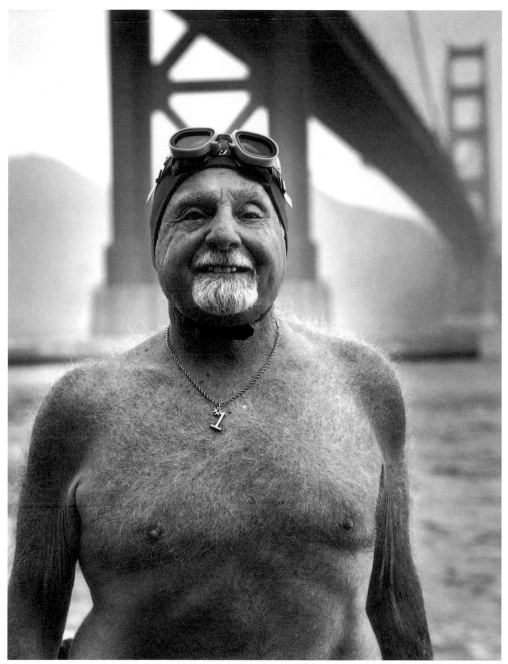

Joe Bruno, age 83

Runner, age 82

Just me, Ada Thomas, approximately ten years older and still deeply in love with myself. I am crazy about this girl, so I continue to use what I got and do the best with what I have. Counting my blessings and giving thanks to God enables me to be like "Old Man River"—keep on rolling along.

—*Ada Thomas*

Ada won the seventy-plus division in the San Francisco Marathon in 1984. She runs every day in Golden Gate Park, where I photographed her. Everybody who walks in the park knows her. As a child, Ada was not allowed to run because, according to her mother, "running was for boys."

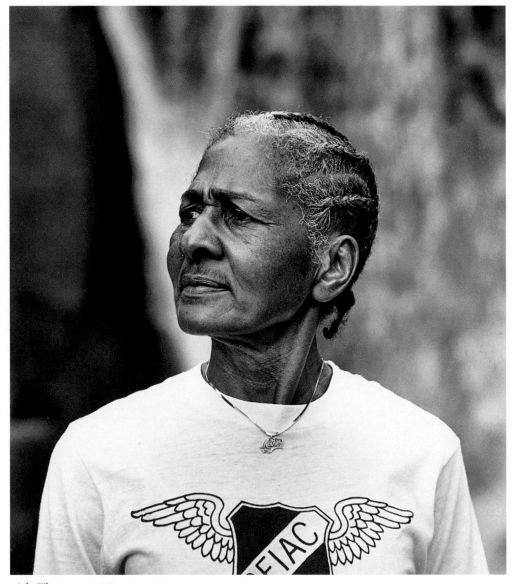

Ada Thomas, age 72

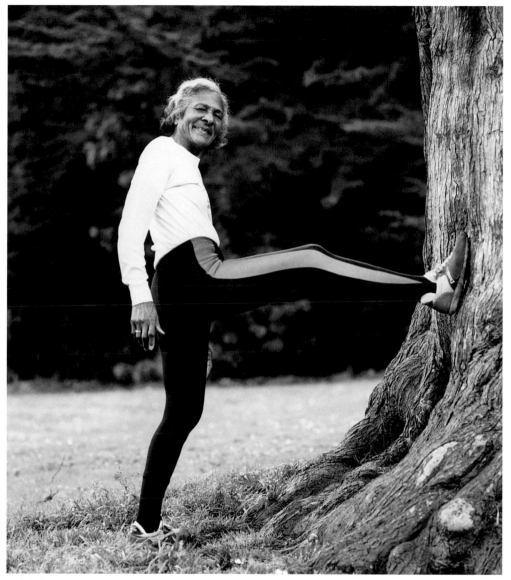

Ada Thomas, age 82

We are all happier in many ways when we are old than when we were young. The young sow wild oats, the old grow sage.

—*Winston Churchill*

"L.O.L."

Fencer, age 77

She's seventy-seven years old. She fences like a demon. And she wants to be known only as the "Little Old Lady." "Just call me 'L.O.L.,'" says this very private lady. "That's it."

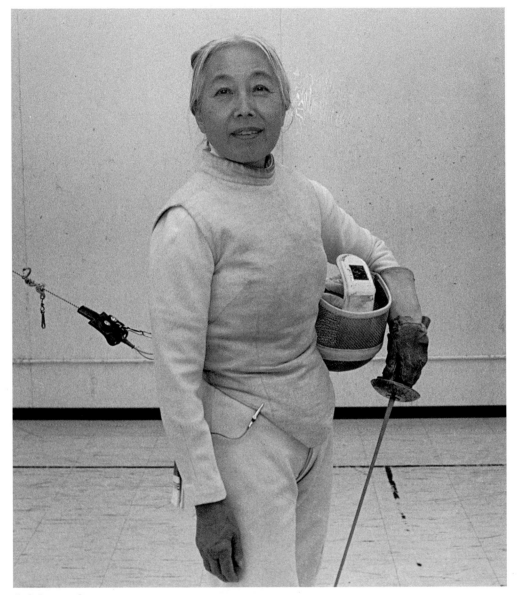

L.O.L., age 67

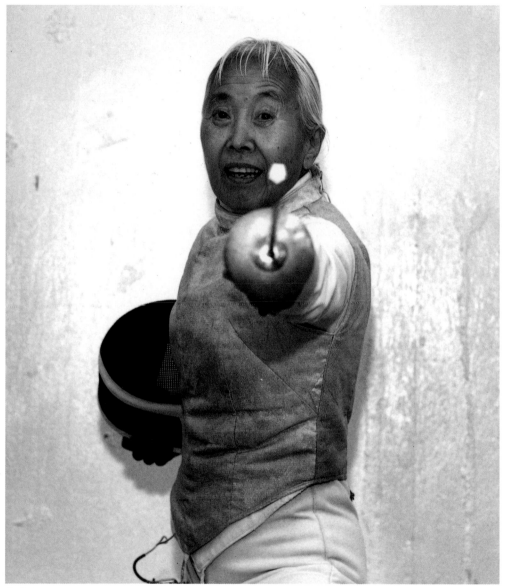

L.O.L., age 77

JOHN TURNER

Weight lifter, age 79

I firmly believe that everybody should exercise as a function of their physical condition, their age, and their condition at the start of their exercise program, which means they should be cleared by a physician to exercise. The exercise should start with something simple like walking. When they can walk two miles, they should then begin to use light weights. But beneath that is the firm belief that exercise is necessary to the full enjoyment of life, body, and mind. Exercise should be properly planned and executed and will benefit, not harm, anyone. Finally, I think that there is no age limit to exercise. Recent research indicates the benefits of weight lifting in people in their seventies, eighties, and even nineties. I hope that exercise at my age fosters physical and mental well-being. It is my profound ambition that by my words and by my actions I can encourage others, young and old, to use and enjoy their bodies.

—*John Turner*

John's perfect workout at this stage in his life is:

> *fifteen minutes of walking*
> *fifteen minutes on the Stairmaster*
> *one hour on weights—the whole body*
> *with free weights.*

He likes to do this three times a week.

8

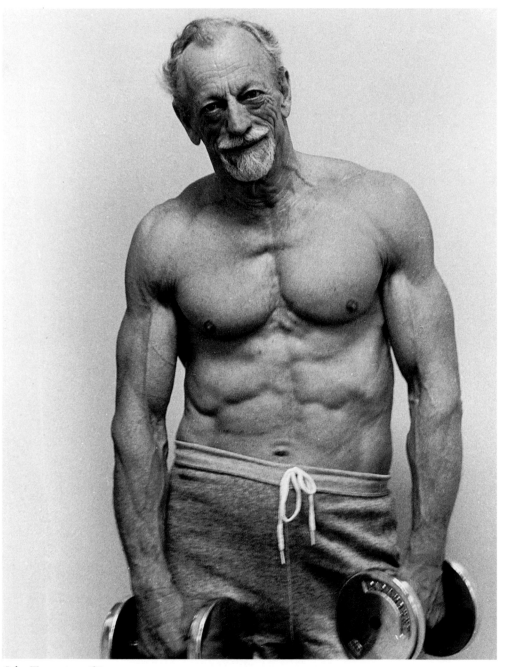

John Turner, age 67

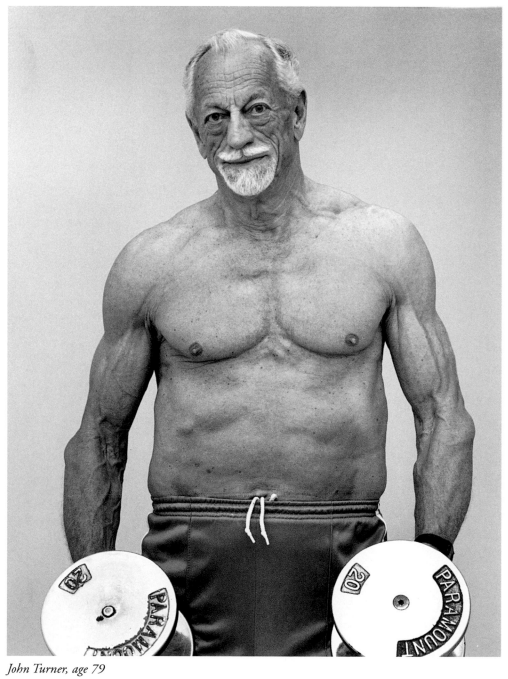

John Turner, age 79

ELS TUINZING

Runner, age 74

Els has slowed down some after a cancer oper-
ation and a total shoulder replacement, but
she still loves to jog the Dipsea Race—a diffi-
cult run of 7.2 miles over coastal hills—and
she rides her bike daily. "Just do it," she says.

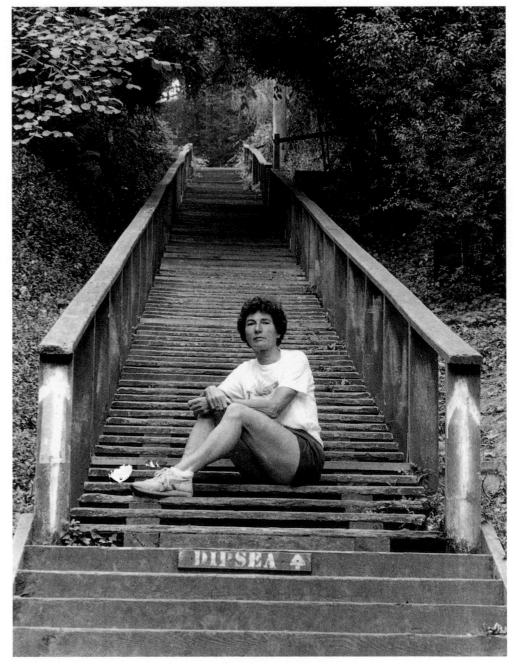

Els Tuinzing, age 61

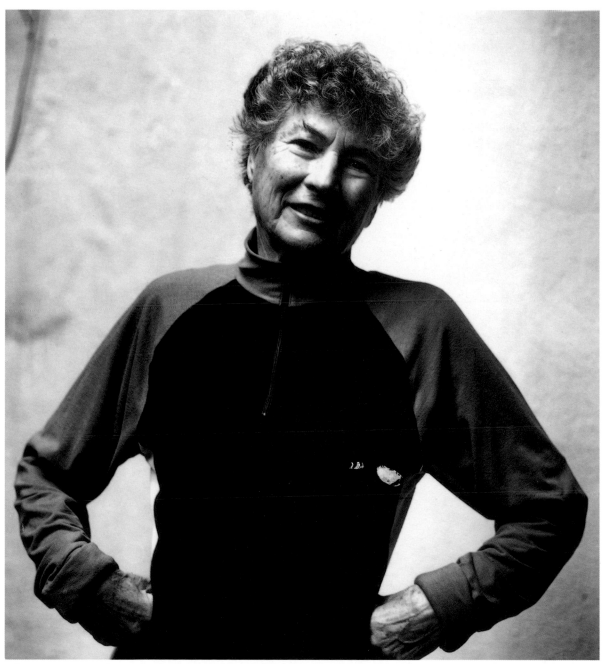

Els Tuinzing, age 74

Trick roper, age 73

Indispensable to any cowboy's daily routine is the rope. This basic tool takes skill—lots of it—and undoubtedly some ropers develop unique methods of handling ropes that eventually become tricks.

—*Kent Diehl*

Kent holds the Guinness world record in international trick and fancy roping for twirling the biggest loop (more than eighty feet in circumference) while lying flat on his back. He takes his trusty lariat with him wherever he goes. "As long as I have my rope," Kent says, laughing, *"I can stand on a corner and rope my way home."*

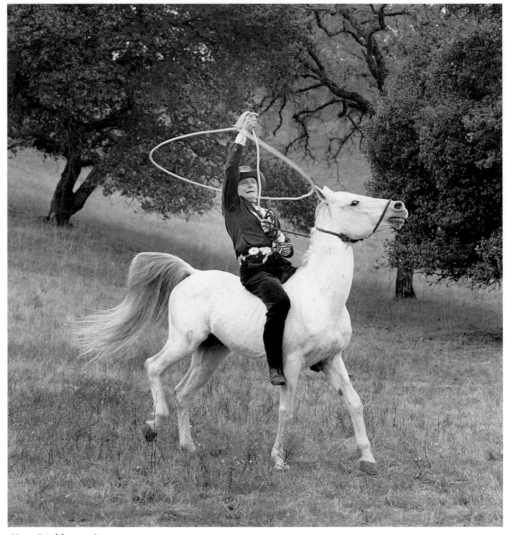

Kent Diehl, age 63

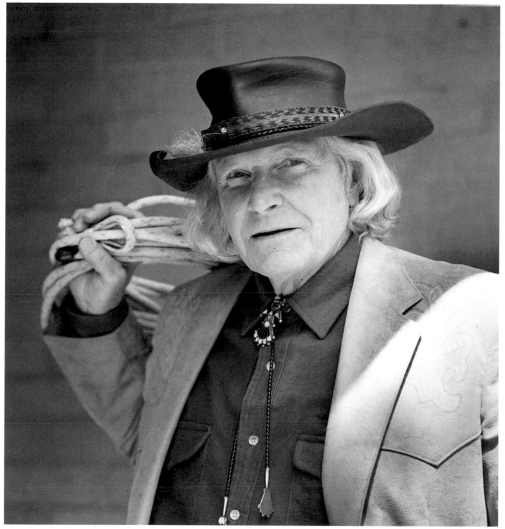

Kent Diehl, age 73

Karate student, age 90

Eleanor is an advanced karate student and a poet (she is a member of the International Poets Society). When I first photographed her ten years ago, she had a purple belt. Now she sports a brown belt, and sometime soon she'll have the black. She hails from South Dakota, where her sisters, ages ninety-six and ninety-eight, live, and describes life around her as very different from her earlier days: "The circus no longer comes to town." Every year she returns to her hometown to visit her family. After one of those visits, she wrote the poem on the opposite page.

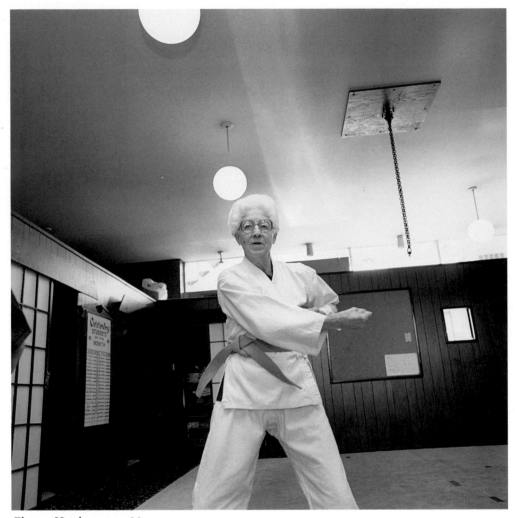

Eleanor Hyndman, age 80

Just one last time to travel back
to where you come from

To walk the old paths through
fields and meadows on your
way to the schoolhouse
of bygone days!

You picture in your mind
the classmates that walked
with you—the teasing—
snowball fights—races—you
come to the school yard
but—sadly the little white
     schoolhouse is gone!

You visit your old hometown
picture in your mind
The "Old Settler's Picnic"
The theater—a dime to
     see a movie!
Not there now—The Chautauqua
does not come each summer—
     The Circus—no more!

One last time you stand
look down the railroad track
The train that blew its steam
whistle as it came to town
is silent—The depot gone!

The old hometown has changed
One last time you visit
     the cemetery
The names on tombstones Oh!
so familiar—too late to
     visit them!

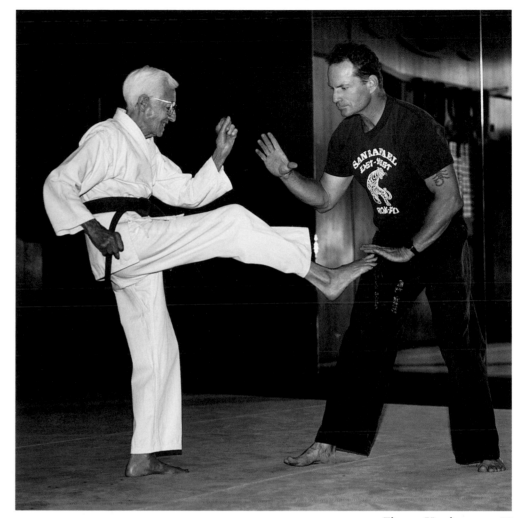

Eleanor Hyndman, age 90

You say a prayer and ask
yourself, "Why did I wait
so long to come home?"
We have only one last time
     Just one last time
     Only one last time
          to say
     "I love you"!

          —*Eleanor Hyndman*

ERNA NEUBAUER

Aerobics instructor, age 86

You can be flexible, active, and attractive at any age. I know from experience because I've been kicking around this playground for eighty-plus years and I still move easily. I feel more into life, more caring about people, and more appreciative of myself than I did forty years ago. The secret is that I keep moving all the time. I have total use of my body. I am going to remind you: The first thing is that we should eat less, not more, and be more careful of what we eat. Keep telling yourself, "I'm not getting older; I'm getting better." We will never again be a terrific twenty, but we can be a fabulous eighty.

—*Erna Neubauer*

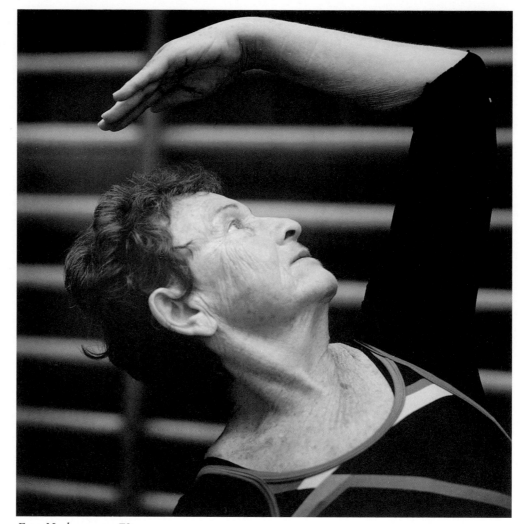

Erna Neubauer, age 73

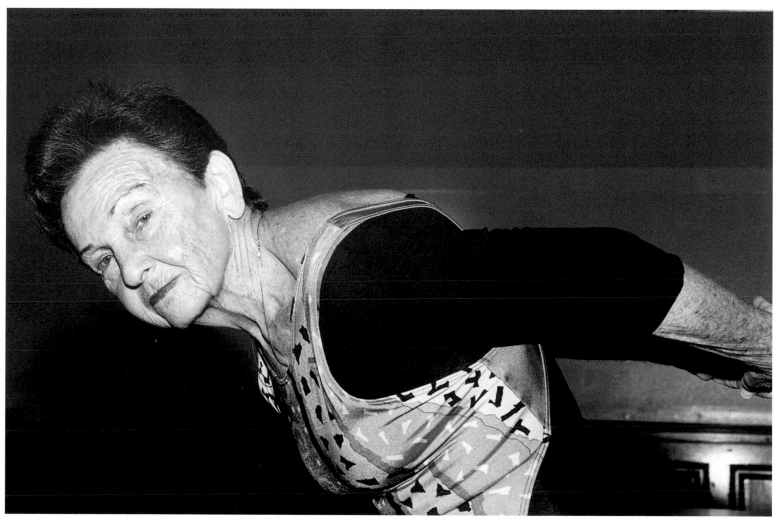

Erna Neubauer, age 86

ANNABEL MARSH

Runner, age 72

In 1984, Annabel was the oldest of three women who ran across the United States—3,261 miles. Their cross-country run celebrated the first women's marathon event in the Olympics, held that year. She has run ninety-six marathons and hopes to complete her hundredth by July 1996.

Annabel is founder of the Peak Busters, an organization that encourages women to run Pikes Peak, a feat that she herself has accomplished twenty times. Her training regimen includes five days of running each week and lots of nonfat yogurt.

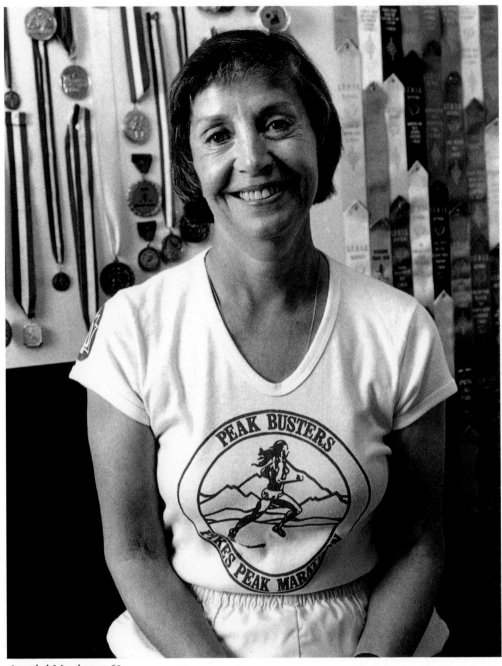

Annabel Marsh, age 60

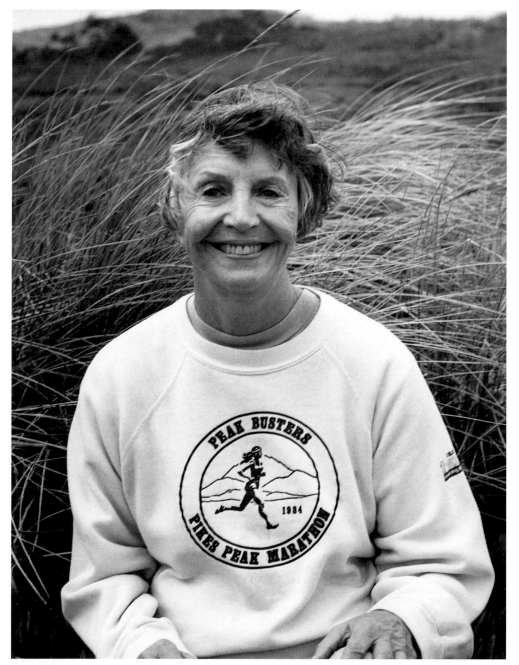

Annabel Marsh, age 72

JIM LEM

Weight lifter, age 67

Jim is a four-time World Master Powerlifting Champion and holds seven world records for his age group. He is the first man over the age of sixty to squat-lift more than 600 pounds.

Twenty-six years ago, at the age of forty-one, Jim saw a photograph of himself forty pounds overweight and was horrified. He took up weight lifting and became a champion. Although he has shown himself to be the best in the world among master competitors, Jim prefers to compete with young lifters because the competition is stiffer. He still has records to set and believes his best is yet to come.

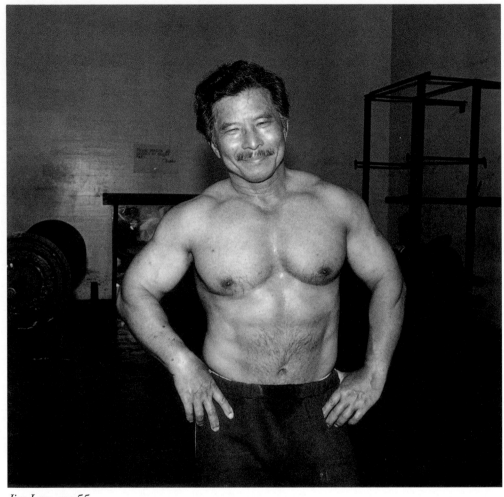

Jim Lem, age 55

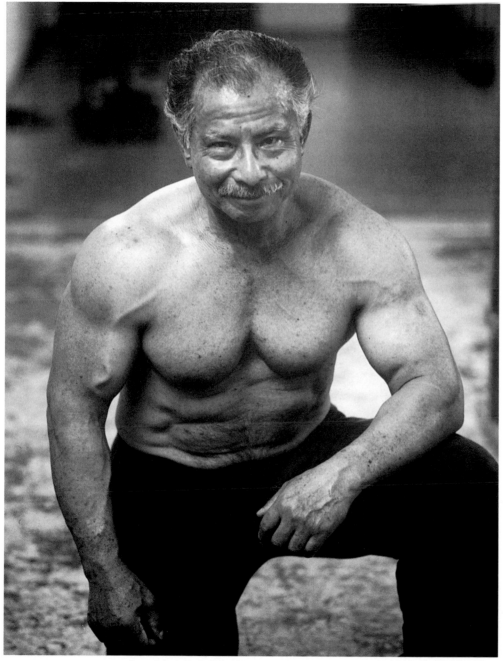

Jim Lem, age 67

LOUIS UHL

Lobsterman, age 86

Three times a week, in winter and summer, Louis violates his doctor's orders by going out on Long Island Sound to recover his lobster pots. A heart attack sixteen years ago hardly slowed him down. His doctor told him to stop lobstering, and he says his aching back agrees. But he cannot resist the call of the lobsters, the salt air, and the sheer physical joy of pulling in his fifty-pound pots and the catch.

Louis lives in his old family house in Branford, Connecticut, and sleeps in the same bed he was born in.

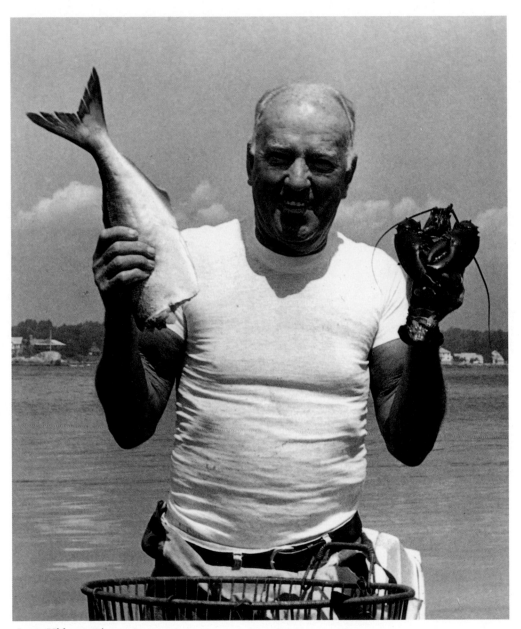

Louis Uhl, age 74

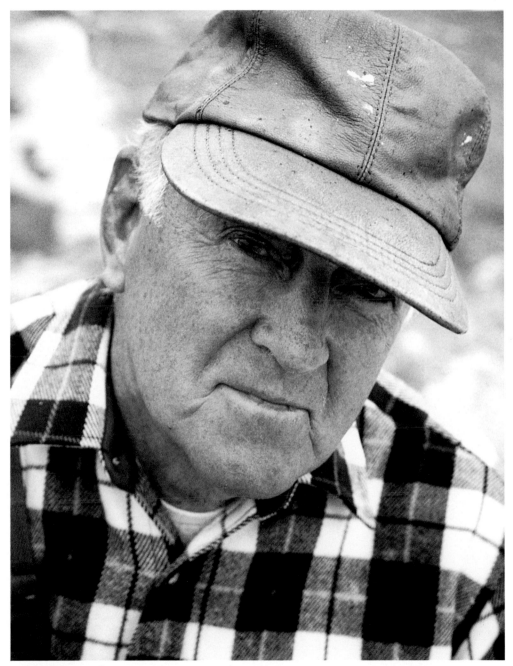

Louis Uhl, age 86

HELEN ZECHMEISTER

Weight lifter, age 91

They called me from Italy last week to compete there, but I was too busy and could not go. The greatest pleasure in my life is my marriage. I have been married sixty-eight years to the same guy, Joseph, and we have done everything together from the moment we met, at a dance at the University of Vienna, Austria. He and my coach, Norman Manoogian, have been my greatest fans.

—*Helen Zechmeister*

At the age of ninety-one, Helen works out three times a week and deadlifts 200 pounds. She is limber enough to do a full split, and she can touch the palms of her hands flat on the floor without bending her knees.

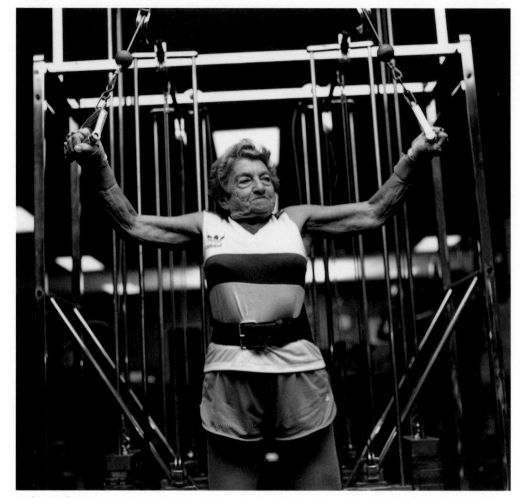

Helen Zechmeister, age 81

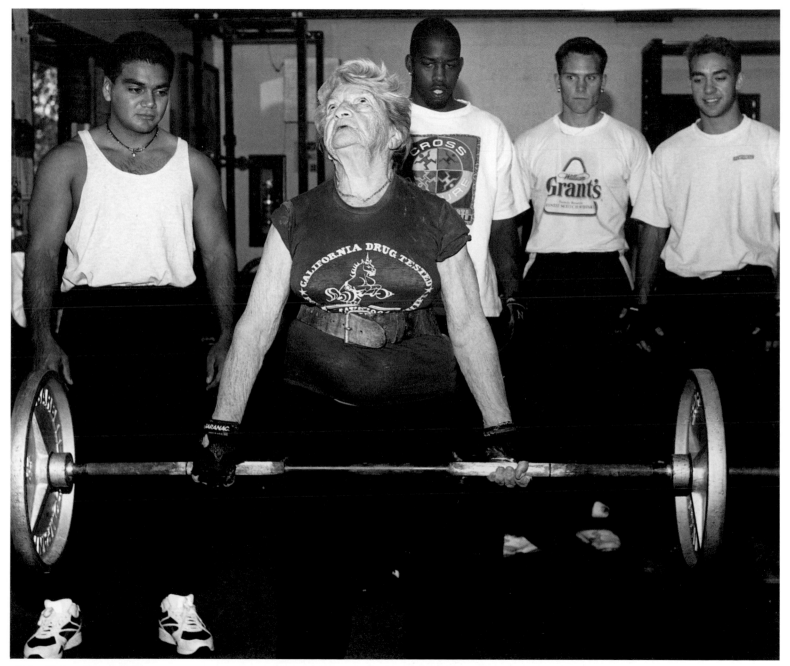

Helen Zechmeister, age 91

JOE ZECHMEISTER

Weight lifter, age 91

Joe is Helen's lifelong companion and work-out partner.

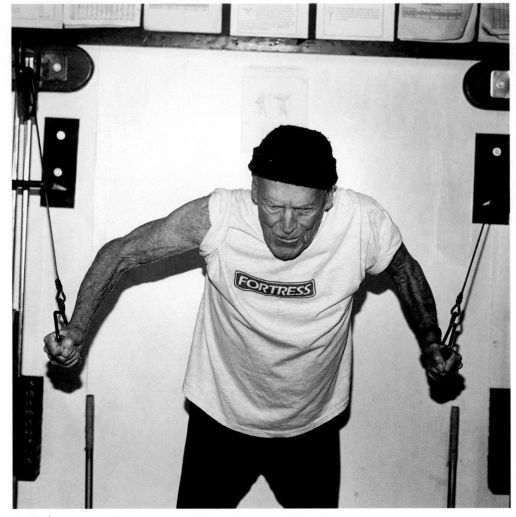

Joe Zechmeister, age 91

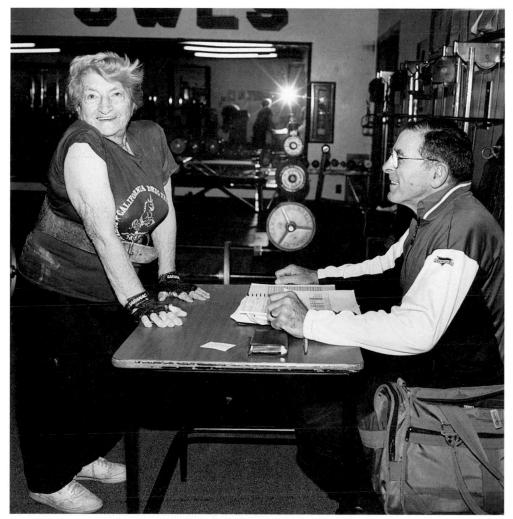

Helen Zechmeister, age 91, with her coach, Norman Manoogian

F. EDWARD
LITTLE AND
MARIE WILCOX-
LITTLE

Swimmers, ages 83 and 73, respectively

When I first met them twelve years ago, Edward and Marie were sweethearts and swim mates and in superb physical condition. They are as trim now as they were in high school and act like young lovers. In 1995, Edward and Marie got married and moved into a new house. Despite their busy lives, they continue to compete in national and international masters swimming meets. They are medalists in freestyle, the butterfly stroke, the backstroke, and the breast stroke.

Ed sent me the poems on the opposite page, one of which he wrote on his eighty-first birthday.

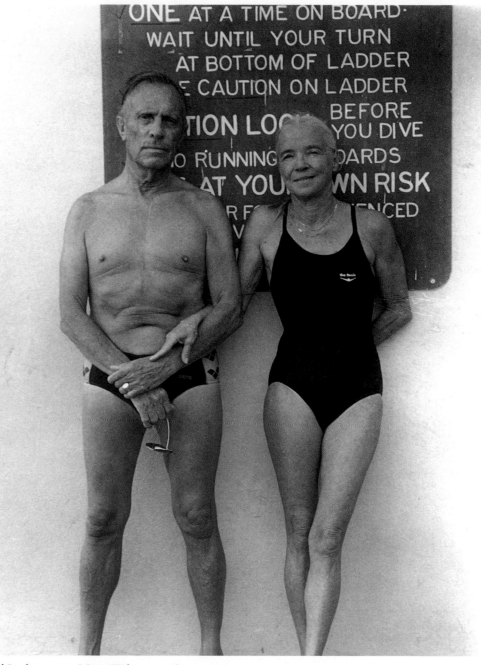

Ed Little, age 71; Marie Wilcox, age 61

SOME REFLECTIONS ON MY EIGHTY-FIRST BIRTHDAY

When you turn eighty, that's a propitious day.
But when you're eighty-one, what can you say?

To what new goals or what new task?
Qué pasa, amigo? you wistfully ask.
You have a thousand things to do
And they all seem exciting and new.

But you are already old. Or so you are told.
So don't worry about getting older than old.

Your plans for this day? Or, for that matter,
    this year?
You have no dues to pay, and no cause for fear.

You might like the year eighty-one, when all is
    said and done.
You have nothing to prove, and you have
    already won.

—F. Edward Little

It would be much less complex
If in the life I live next,
God borns me rich—and undersexed.

—F. Edward Little

So, if you are planning to *live* in your eighties, what do you do? What would you do if you had a beautiful sweetheart and felt that you might have missed a few things in the rapid scramble to octogenaria? Well, you could get married, take a honeymoon cruise, buy a new sports car, purchase a lovely home, become proficient in the expanding computer magic . . .

Following this line of thinking, in the past year Marie and I were married in a gorgeous formal wedding. We took a honeymoon cruise. We bought a new car. We have just moved into our new home on a golf course. We are right on schedule, except for one thing: I am lagging a bit in my computer abilities. We may just drop that item. After all, when you reach eighty, you have to give up a few things.

—*F. Edward Little*

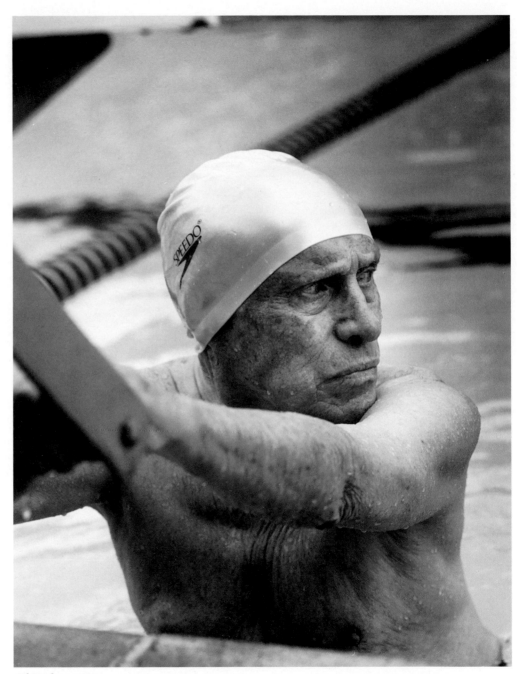

Ed Little, age 83

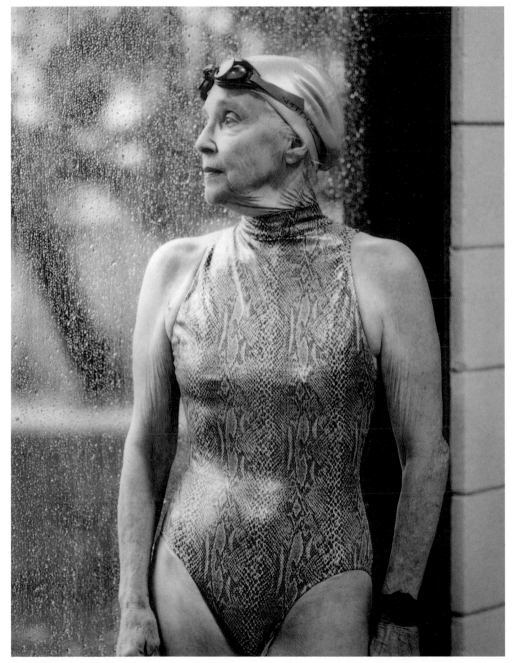

Marie Wilcox-Little, age 73

Literature has neglected the old and their emotions. The novelists never told us that in life, as in other matters, the young are just beginners and that the art of loving matures with age and experience.

—*Isaac Bashevis Singer*

NED SHUTKIN

Weight lifter, age 84

At a vigorous eighty-four, my stepfather is a modern-day Renaissance man and an inspiration to everyone who knows him. A retired orthopedic surgeon at Yale University Hospital, he is a busy medical consultant, a writer, a raconteur, and a student of history and literature. He keeps in shape by pumping iron and working out on his Minimax.

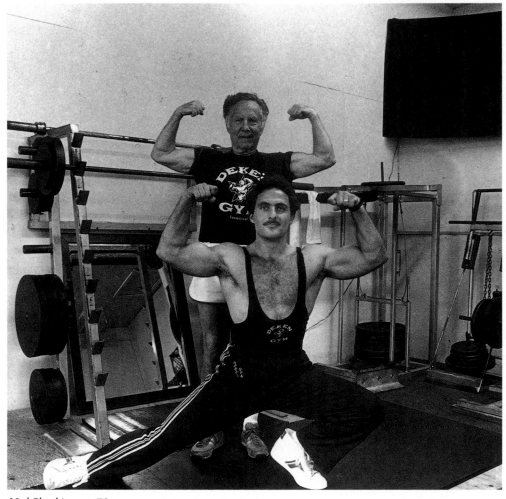

Ned Shutkin, age 72

Ned has a wonderful knack for limericks.
Here are a few samples.

In Connecticut I'm now called an old fossil,
A description I don't find colossal.
The "fossil" I don't mind;
It's the "old" that's unkind—
But maybe that's what makes me docile.

The golden years are a myth;
There's always something you're with.
It can be cardiac disease
Or an asthmatic wheeze;
One is constantly badgered forthwith.

Anacreon, a Greek poet of old
Never would do what he was told.
He would much sooner
Act like a junior
And remain feisty and bold.

People consider old age a curse;
Of that there is no opinion diverse.
But whatever is thought
The thinking is fraught
With the knowledge that the alternative's
    worse.

Men worry about cholesterol;
Women worry about stilbestrol.
But this very worry
Makes them age in a hurry;
It would be better if they ignored them all.

—*Ned Shutkin*

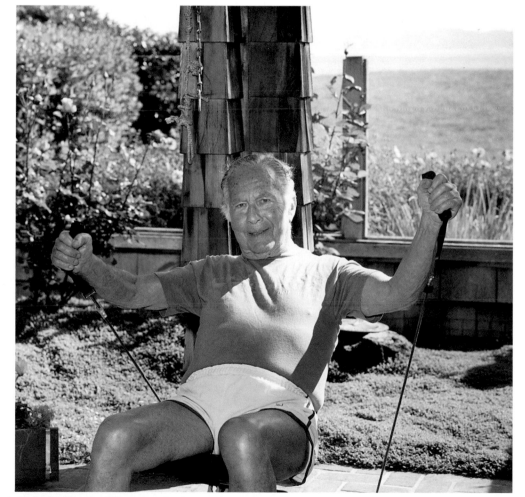

Ned Shutkin, age 84

Skier, scuba diver, and equestrian, age 75

Mary is my mother and my best friend. She grew up in Germany, had me, and dodged bombs in World War II before coming to America. Now she is a California girl who enjoys skiing in the Rockies, scuba diving in the Caribbean, and riding to the hounds in Connecticut. She loves the outdoors and the fun of sports. "I never pursue a sport just for the exercise," she says. "I play strictly for the enjoyment and for an adrenalin rush." Her advice on keeping a youthful appearance: "Don't wear your glasses when you look in the mirror."

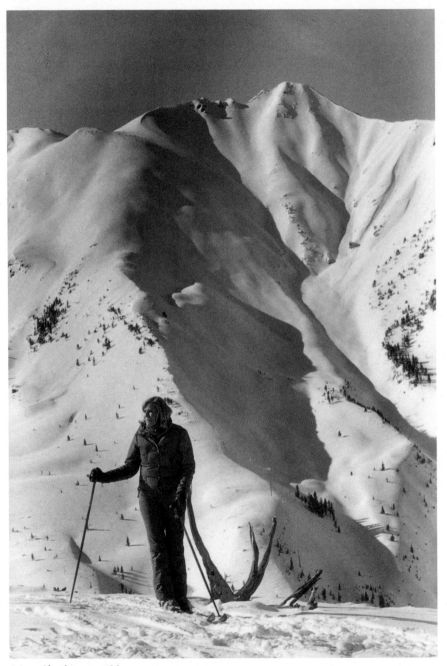

Mary Shutkin, age 64

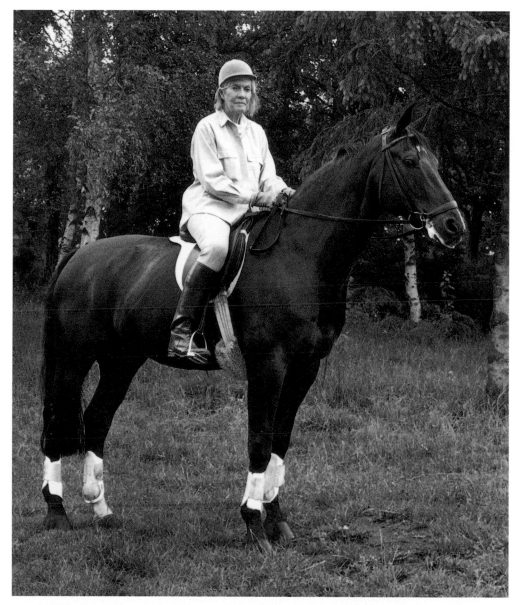

Mary Shutkin, age 75

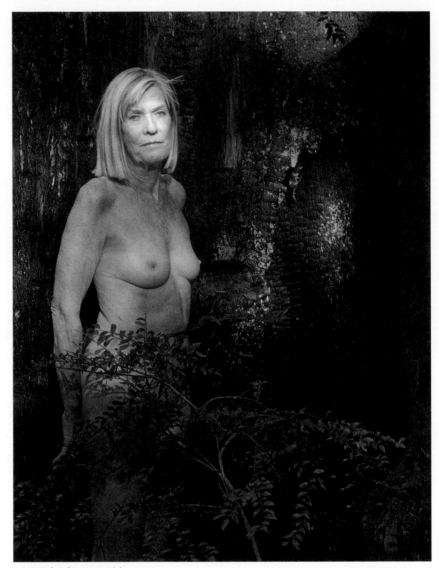

Mary Shutkin, age 64

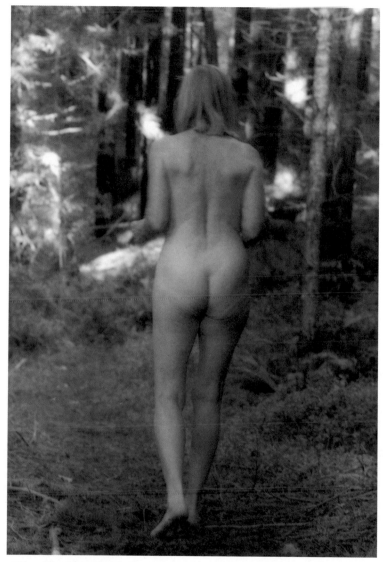

Mary Shutkin, age 75

Mary's long-suffering husband, Ned (see pages 32–33), offered this limerick as a tribute to her.

The woman is Teutonic,
The woman bionic.
She has a whim of iron.
She spent the war years in Bayern.
Skis down the course,
Jumps with the horse.

—*Ned Shutkin*

And, Ned notes,

In the first edition she was the centerfold;
In the second edition she is not so bold.

ULYSSES

Come, my friends,
'Tis not too late to seek a newer world.
Push off, and sitting well in order smite
The sounding furrows; for my purpose holds
To sail beyond the sunset, and the baths
Of all the western stars, until I die.
It may be that the gulfs will wash us down;
It may be we shall touch the Happy Isles,
And see the great Achilles, whom we knew.
Though much is taken, much abides; and though
We are not now the strength which in old days
Moved earth and heaven, that which we are we are.
One equal temper of heroic hearts,
Made weak by time and fate, but strong in will
To strive, to seek, to find, and not to yield.

—Alfred, Lord Tennyson

PHYLLIS "FLAME FOLLY" MARCUS

Clown, dancer, and singer, age 70

Phyllis is a bighearted professional clown who loves to entertain in hospitals and convalescent homes under her stage name, Flame Folly. She has overcome a number of serious ailments and understands how important laughter can be to people in pain.

When I first met Phyllis, she was performing a song-and-dance routine in a convalescent home. She was full of life, laughter, and a little mischief, and the audience loved her.

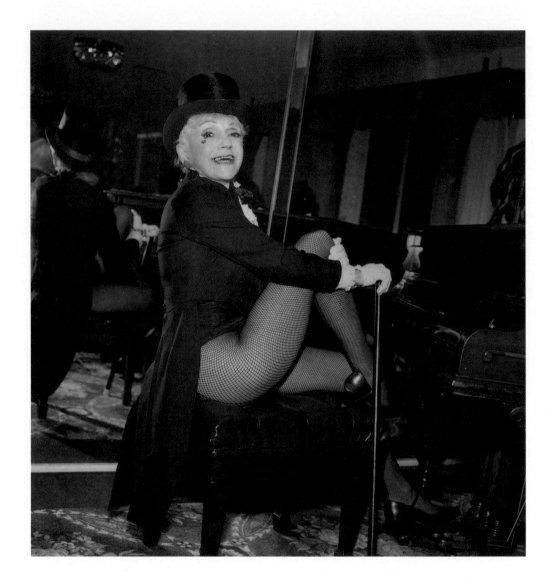

ROSE SCHWARTZ

Dancer, age 94

I am most fortunate that I have been able to make a good living dancing. I think God's greatest gift to humanity is music, and the next is the ability to move to music. From the time I saw my first dance at age nine, I knew that I must dance. At age ninety-four, I am still teaching dance to seniors.

—*Rose Schwartz*

Rose dances and teaches every day. Some of her classes have as many as 200 older students.

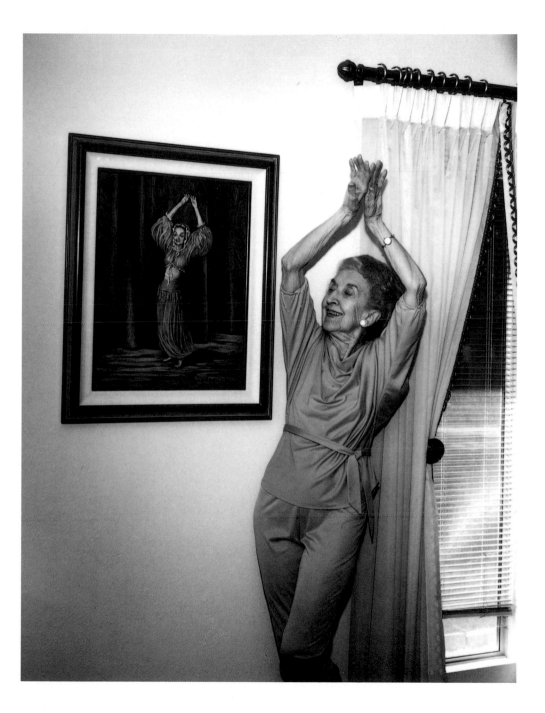

GEORGE McGINNIS

Track and field athlete, age 61

There is no need to find a rocking chair after age sixty. You can enjoy the sports and events you have always enjoyed, but at a different pace. It's heartwarming to see people in their seventies, eighties, and nineties competing in these types of events. There was a 100-meter sprinter in Columbus who was ninety-five. His performance was one of the greatest sights I have ever seen.

—*George McGinnis*

George is the national shot put champion in his age category.

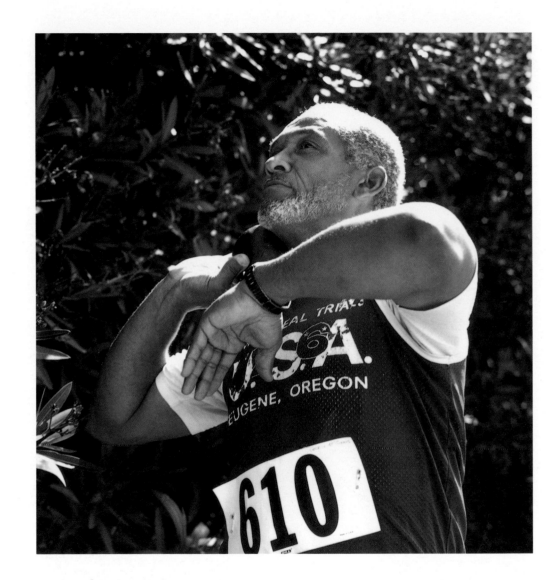

SHIRLEY DIETDERICH

Track and field athlete, age 69

Long after the age at which most athletes hang up their cleats and retire, Shirley was just beginning her career as a world-class track and field athlete. She started at age forty-eight and has been going full steam ever since. Her most recent accomplishment was winning a gold medal with the women's 4 x 100-meter relay team at the World Masters Championships in Miyazaki, Japan, in the sixty-five to sixty-nine age group.

Shirley is a competitor in the 100- and 200-meter events and a javelin and discus thrower. In 1994 she placed first in the nationals in the discus in Eugene, Oregon. She runs six days a week, lifts weights two to three times a week, and swims and throws twice a week.

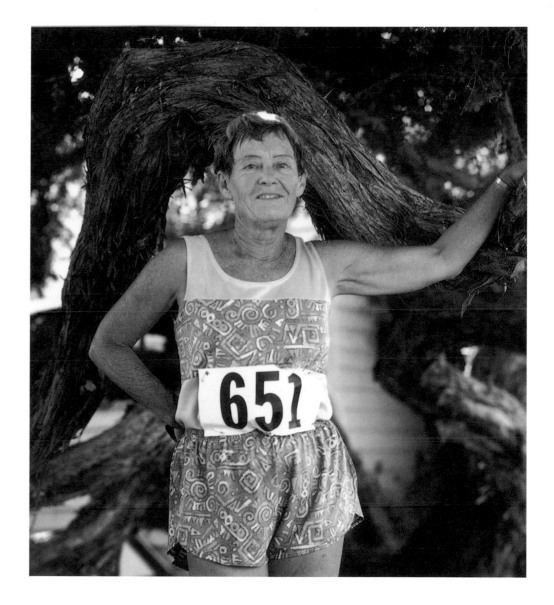

SUN CITY
STEPPERS

Dancers, average age 70

Pictured here are the advanced tap dancers from Sun City, Arizona, with their teacher, Norma Jean Denny. They practice five days a week and have a ball.

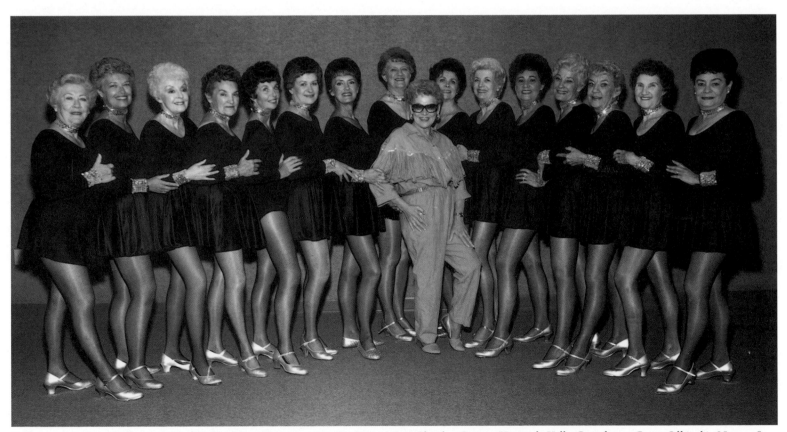

Left to right: Geri Hoffman, Gitta Cryder, Mary Nauman, Juanita Devers, Peg Chaplo, Connie Howard, Kelly Greenburg, Grace Olbinski, Norma Jean Denny (center front), Jane Marter, Ann Yacyshyn, Jean Wohlfeill, Yvonne Paullus, Pat Armor, Gladys Bielawa, Jerry Bland

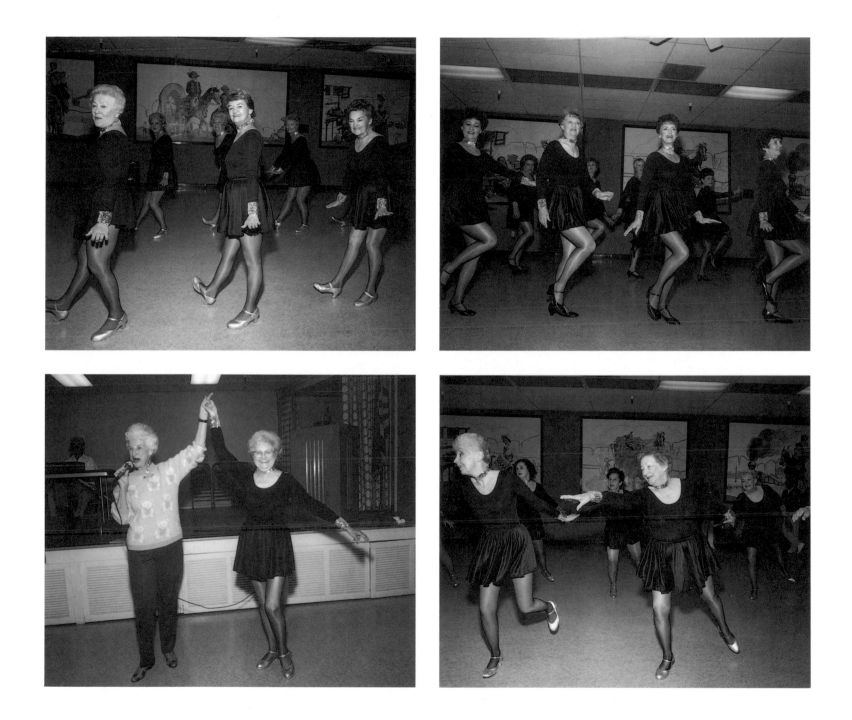

JAE HOWELL

Swimmer, age 73

After operating my swim school for thirty-five years, teaching approximately 1,000 students a year, I finally retired with no thought of involving myself in the swim world. When a friend suggested I go to a masters meet to watch her compete, I decided to go the whole way—and enter. Since then it's been an exciting world of new friends, travel, and being mentioned as an inspiration to several people.

—*Jae Howell*

The only problem Jae mentioned after I sent her this picture was this: "Swimmers are definitely at a disadvantage when it comes to pictures, particularly at a meet. Soaked hair, no makeup, sun-dried skin, and red-streaked eyes are the 'minuses.'" Jae has been an All-American swimmer for the past five years (which means that she has earned the fastest times in the United States in her events). Last year she received ten "firsts" in her age group. Age groups are divided into five-year increments, which actually makes swimmers look forward to growing older.

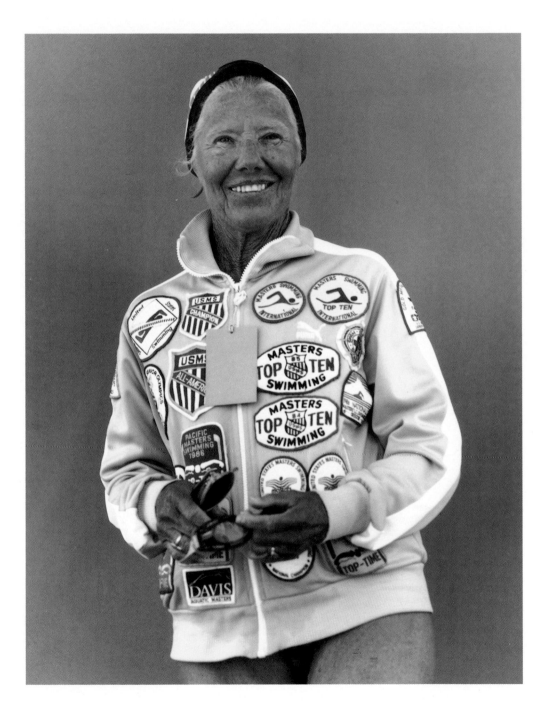

BILL JOHNSON

Swimmer, age 77

Bill Johnson is a burly, white-bearded guy who is full of life and loves to lecture anyone who will listen to him about the tremendous benefits of remaining physically active as one grows older. He is a good example of his own advice and has been among the top ten masters swimmers in the country for the past twenty-one years.

Bill tried open-ocean swimming in Santa Cruz in 1938 but found the water too cold. He tried it again a half century later, in 1988. Still too cold. He promises one more try, in 2038.

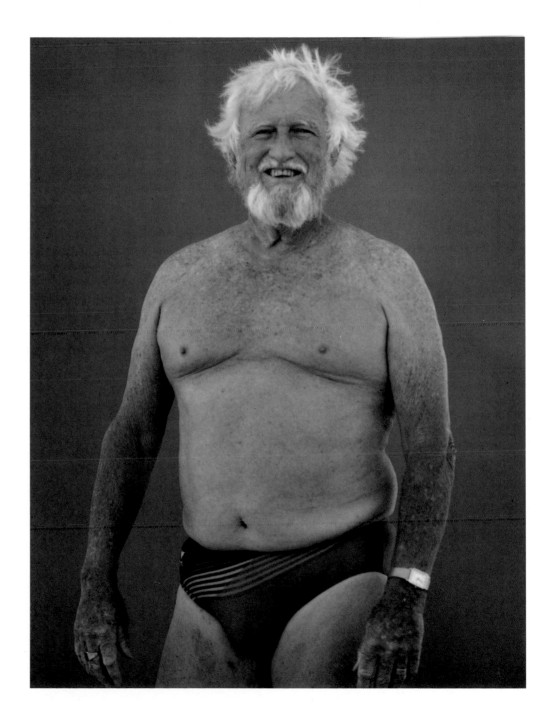

JERRY SILSDORF

Track and field athlete, age 72

Jerry is on the board of directors of the California State Senior Games Committee. He competes nationally and internationally and has the following on his business card:

Over 50???

You are not alone . . . Just one of

63 MILLION AMERICANS!

That is the WEALTHIEST GROUP in the

Whole Nation!

The total combined group income is

OVER 800 BILLION DOLLARS

A further look shows the following:

77% of U.S. FINANCIAL ASSETS

HALF THE DISCRETIONARY INCOME

40% OF ALL CONSUMER DEMAND

NICE GROUP

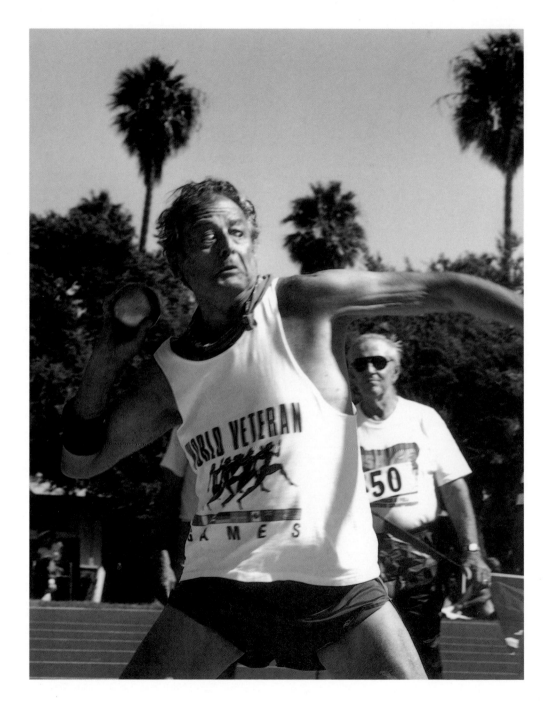

JIM SULLENGER

Track and field athlete, age 75

During a Thanksgiving dinner in 1990, the conversation turned to sports and Jim reminisced about his prowess with the discus and shot put during his high school days. Two days later, he received a discus in the mail from a dinner companion and launched his second career as a track and field athlete. Now, at the age of seventy-five, he is a regular competitor in masters track and field competitions. In 1994 he took a silver medal at the national masters track and field meet in Eugene, Oregon.

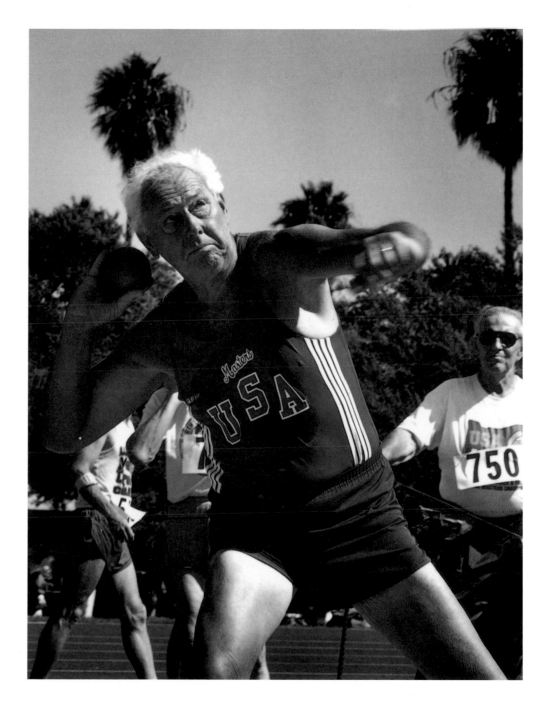

DICK ELTON

Hiker and mountaineer, age 78

If you were to take a photograph of me, it should probably be of my legs instead of my face. It had never entered my head, but about ten years ago it became very obvious to me that people thought my legs looked pretty good. I give a lot of talks, and about four years ago I was presenting a lesson on backpacking to a group of Girl Scouts. I was grandly dressed in my backpacking costume, explaining in the most interesting manner about clothing, tents, foods, water purification, safety, and the like. Deciding that I should stop and assess how it was all going over, I paused and asked, "Well, does anyone have any questions?" One girl raised her hand and asked, "How can we get a pair of legs like yours?"

—*Dick Elton*

Dick has climbed the highest mountain peaks in each of the forty-eight contiguous states.

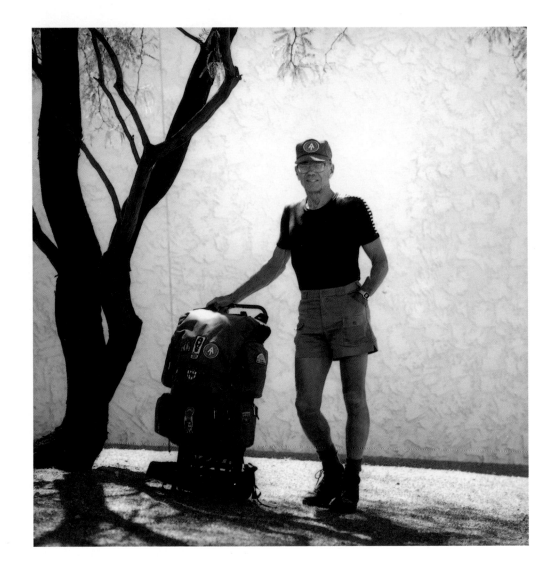

MARIO J. CIAMPI

Tennis player, age 88

As children of the universe, we experience the energy of harmonic action and the vibrations of irreversible change. It is that endless search for balance of the body and the spirit that directs our judgment to live within the demands of the natural law. This pursuit of enlightenment, enriching our sensory world, fulfilling our aspirations, is implemented through our perceptions of love and beauty. This continuous regeneration of life is my vision of aging.

—*Mario J. Ciampi*

Architecture and city planning are Mario's professional pursuits. He also is very involved in cosmic energy research and holistic health programs. He writes: "As we approach the new millennium, our responsibility is to live by the natural law: First we must heal ourselves, then the planet will naturally be healed."

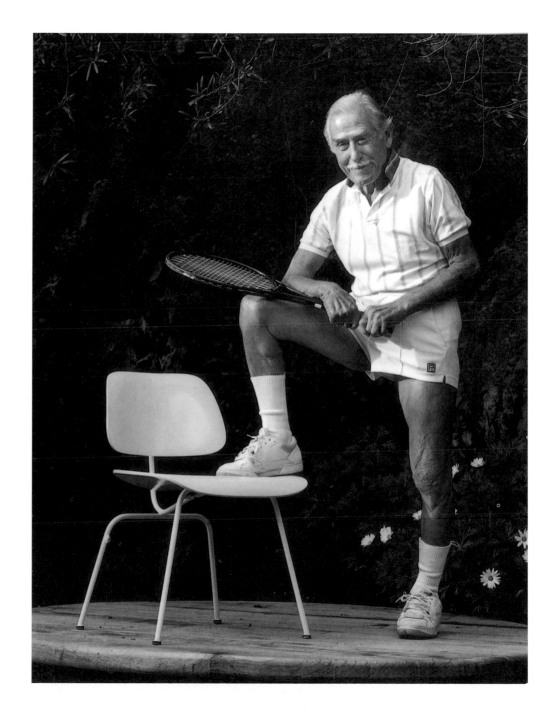

JIM LAW

Sprinter, age 69

Not many years ago I was an overweight, chain-smoking fast-food junkie with a serious cholesterol problem that I didn't know about. I believe that I live today because I joined Senior Games and became the beneficiary of interventions that followed that joining. Principally, those interventions involved a radical shift in diet and the substitution of regular exercise for my forty years of sedentary existence. After seven months of practicing faithfully this new regimen—and it was not simply exercise tacked onto a new diet but a genuine lifestyle change—I lost about twenty-five pounds and my cholesterol reading moved from 322 to 188. In another year or so, I was able to give up my forty-nine-year habit of smoking cigarettes. As a result of these changes, I felt better, looked better, and had less stress and more energy. I was more productive, and life was more fun.

—*Jim Law*

Jim holds six National Senior Olympic records—for the 100-, 200-, and 400-meter sprints.

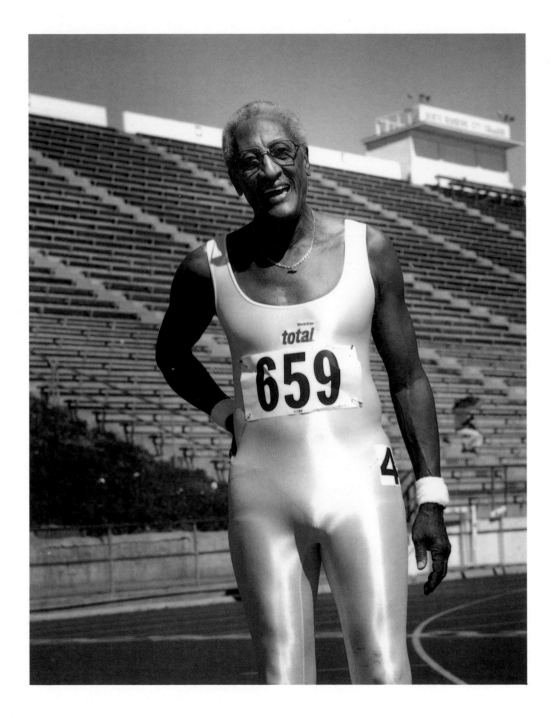

NICK NEWTON

Track and field athlete, age 61

Nick started competing on the masters track circuit twenty-one years ago, when he discovered he had a natural knack for high jumping and sprinting. About fifteen years ago he had a bout with testicular cancer, but he came through the ordeal and is tougher for the experience. In 1994 he took a silver medal in the high jump and the 100-meter event in the Masters Track World Games. He is pictured here at the Santa Barbara masters track meet with his old pal and competitor, Jim Law, after Nick won the 100-yard dash. Jim came in a close second.

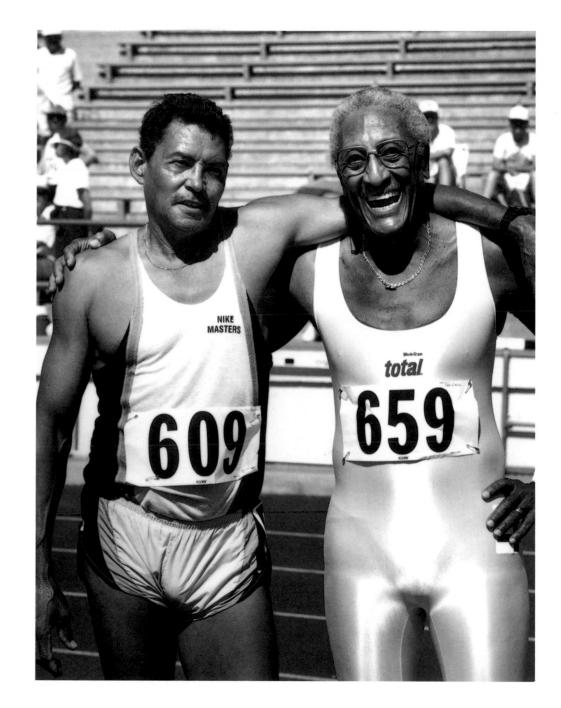

WOODBRIDGE R. "WOODY" BROWN

Surfer, age 83

All my life I wanted to know: Where did I come from, where am I going, and what am I here for? But I never got the answers. Flying and surfing were a welcome rest from these nagging worries. Finally I did what Jesus said to do: "Love and forgive your enemies." And then all the answers came to me.

—*Woody Brown*

Woody is a vigorous old guy who has developed his own unique blend of spirituality and sports that has made him a surfing legend in his home waters at Kahului, Maui, Hawaii. When he launches his giant surfboard, other surfers make way and watch with awe as he rides the heavies.

Woody's training regimen: early to bed, and a firm prohibition against candy, soda pop, drugs, tobacco, and alcohol. He is a vegetarian and tries not to overindulge in sex.

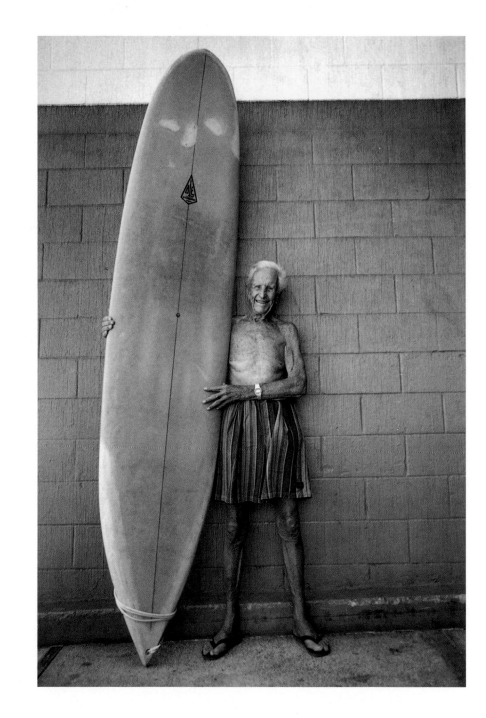

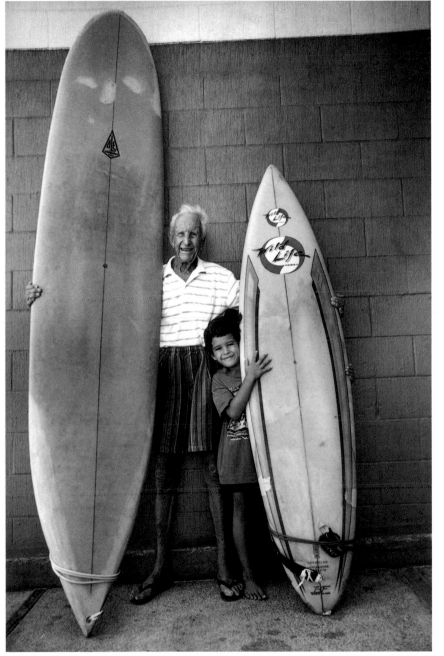

Woody Brown, age 83, and Woody Jr., age 6

YOUTHFUL AGE

Young men dancing, and the old
Sporting I with joy behold;
But an old man gay and free
Dancing most I love to see;
Age and youth alike he shares
For his heart belies his hairs.

—*translated by Thomas Stanley*

JOE BURKE

Boxer, age 62

Five days a week, Joe spars with fighters one-third his age. He has been boxing since the age of sixteen, and even at sixty-two Joe is a formidable presence in the ring. His advice to up-and-coming young pugilists: "Keep swinging; you're always dangerous when you're swinging. Don't sweat the little things—and they all are little things."

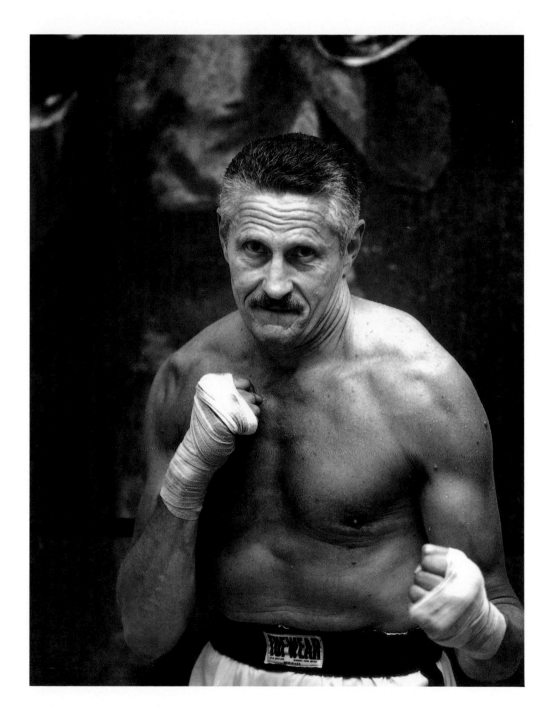

Long-distance runner, age 76

After a lifetime of pills, pot, alcohol, and poor eating habits, I finally wound up in the alcoholic ward at the VA hospital in Palo Alto, California, in 1977. I weighed 235 pounds, and my liver was the size of a football. I was also smoking two to three packs of cigarettes a day. I was so short of breath that I could not climb two flights of stairs without stopping halfway up to catch my breath.

My diagnosis at the VA was acute alcoholism, with a fifty-fifty chance of recovery due to my damaged liver. I realized that this was my last chance to pull my life together. Starting at ground zero, I joined AA and managed to stay sober and feel better long enough to realize that God had given me the one last chance that I had prayed so hard for. However, even though I was not drinking, I was still smoking heavily, drinking ten to fifteen cups of coffee a day, and sleeping poorly. I was sober, and that was all that counted, but I was wondering how long I could hang on.

Then one day I got a book in the mail —*The Complete Book of Running* by Jim Fixx. I read the book from cover to cover and figured it was worth a try to get out there and see if I could become a runner. I went out the next day, April 2, 1978, and I've been running ever since.

I soon became able to run in 10K races,

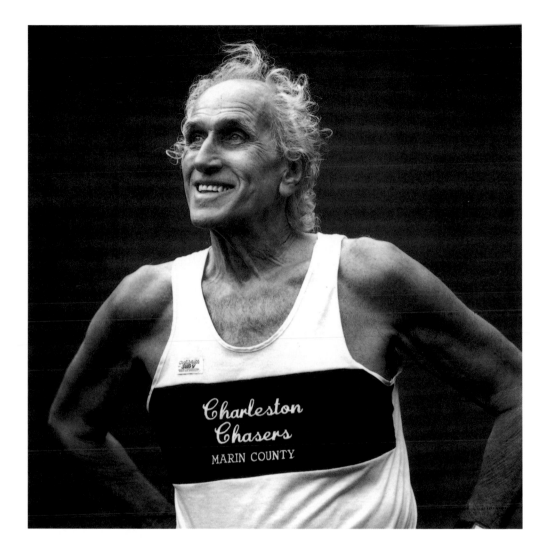

but it was years before I could run the Dipsea Race and the San Francisco Marathon, both of which I ran in 1986. That was the turning point in my life. I felt that if I could run both races and finish in fairly good time, I could do anything! Running is my life, because running gave me life.

—*Fred Ullner*

I saw Fred running in the city where I live. He had headphones on and seemed to be bopping with the music.

PHIL ARNOT

Runner and hiker, age 70

Running has been the rule of my life. It confirms my aliveness and is my Fountain of Youth.

—*Phil Arnot*

Before his recent knee surgery, runner and hiker Phil Arnot ran four miles four or five times a week. Now he's using the Stairmaster and running shorter distances uphill. The 1950 half-mile record holder at UCLA, Phil likes to climb mountains and has conquered 275 of them, including Mt. McKinley. He also leads several wilderness trips through Alaska and the Sierra Nevada each year.

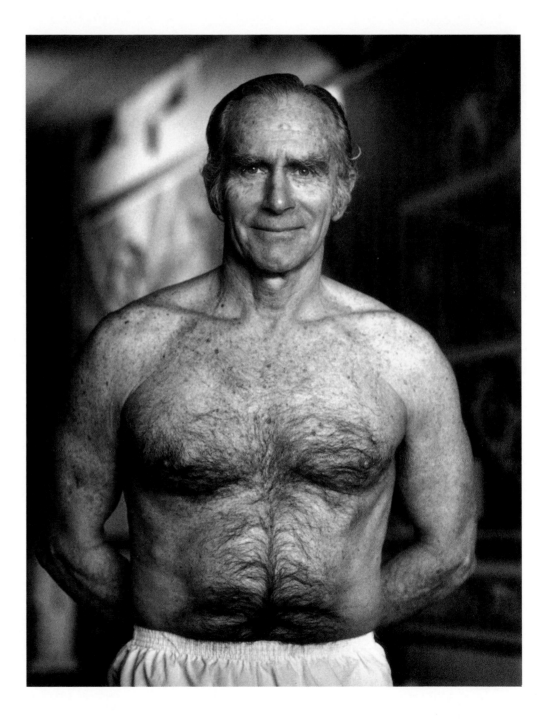

JERRY BALDWIN

Cross-country ski racer, age 77

When I first saw Jerry, he was racing through the streets of San Francisco with roller skis on his feet and ski poles in hand. A serious cross-country skier, Jerry trains during the summer months by roller skiing hundreds of miles a week. He has won many cross-country ski races in the past forty-five years. One of his favorites is the thirty-kilometer Citizens Race in Yosemite, California, in which he has won several gold medals.

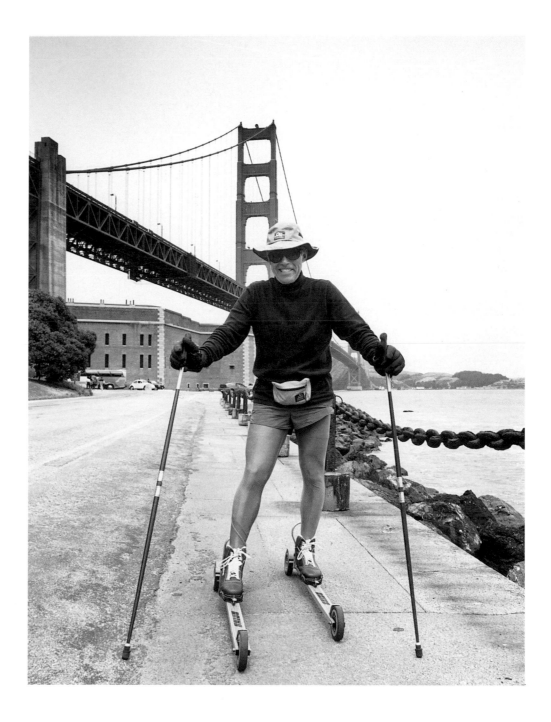

BOB "OLE" OLSON

Surfer, age 66

I like building surfboards, and I love surfing. I am trying to keep the stress level low and stay healthy, so I can continue to surf and shape surfboards.

—*Ole Olson*

Ole's surfboards are famous among surfers. Even our cover boy has one.

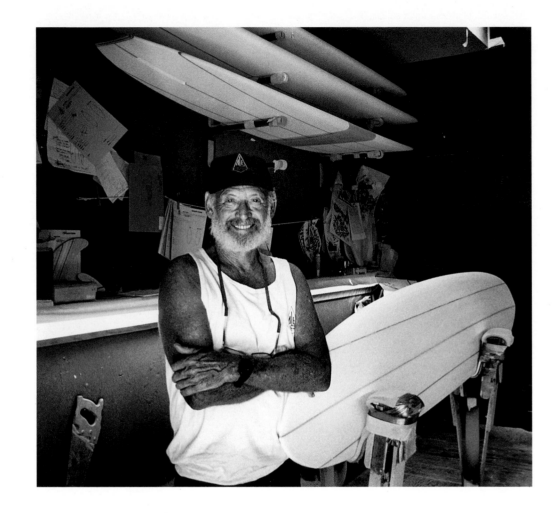

JACK BRAY

Race walker, age 61

Five years ago Jack became a race walker when, nineteen miles into the San Francisco Marathon, he hit the wall. "I was in pain, and I could hardly move," says Jack. "So I started walking very slowly, and alongside of me comes this man race walking and singing and saying 'Good morning.' I tried to keep up with him, but he flew by me. He was Marco Evoniuk, the Olympian."

Jack has become the fastest walker in the world for his age class, winning the five-kilometer walk at the 1995 World Veterans Games. His time was twenty-five minutes, nine seconds.

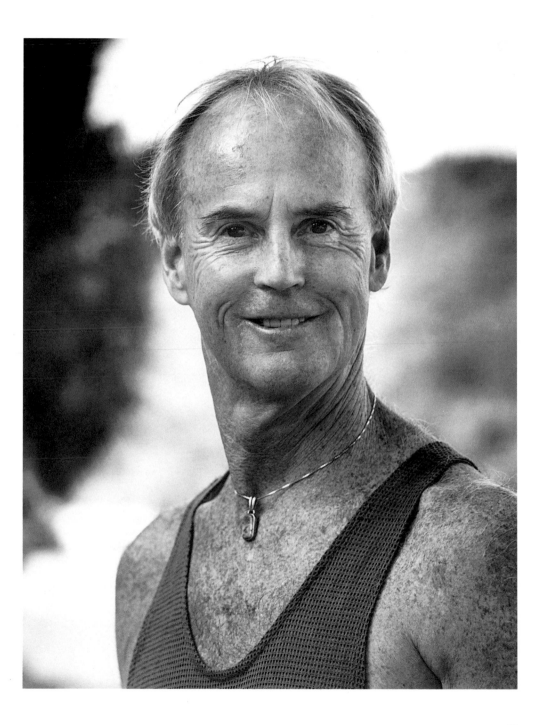

Race walker, age 75

Prior to March 1986, I was known as the "bionic grandfather," who would live to be one hundred and twenty-five. Wanting to study the cello at an early age, I found my priorities ahead of music encompassing sports and politics, which absorbed all of my spare time. Marriage, a child (now age fifty-two) and a grandchild, and more marriages all followed pell-mell as time passed. Suddenly, at age sixty-six, lo and behold, a quadruple bypass! What have we here?

The process of rebuilding my traumatized body involved a step-by-step regimen of walking that eventually evolved into race walking, the healthiest of all aerobic sports. I also felt it vital to lend support to other patients and organized the Marin County, California, chapter of Mended Hearts for that purpose. At the grand age of seventy-two, I became interested in competitive race walking. I have acquired a collection of gold, silver, and bronze medals in the seventy to seventy-four category, and now, at the age of seventy-five, I have become known as the "bionic great grandfather."

—Herm Arrow

Herm Arrow, age 75, and Dorothy Roberts, age 85, in Jack Bray's race walking class

DOROTHY ROBERTS

Race walker, age 85

A couple of years ago Dorothy was sitting around at home, aching with arthritis and feeling her age. It was about that time that she made the big decision to "wear out instead of rust out." She started on a modest walking regimen that turned into a passion for competitive racing. As of the summer of 1995, Dorothy was working out in preparation for the World Masters Games on the East Coast, her heart set on a gold medal.

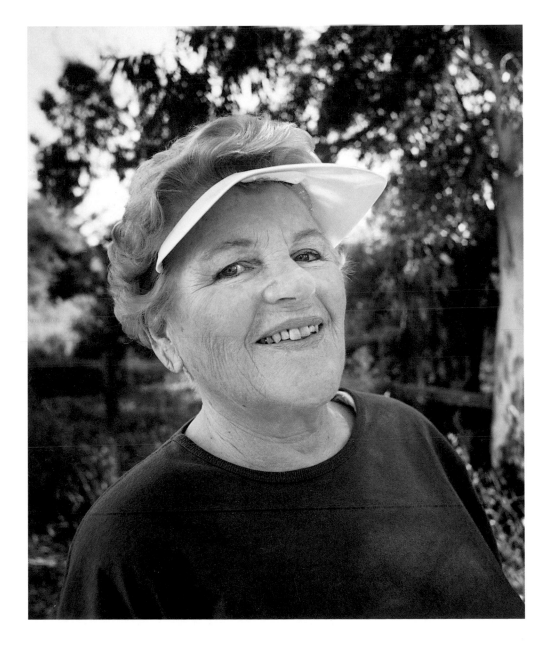

VILLA MARIN
PADDLE TENNIS
TEAM MEMBERS

Average age: 83

An injured knee compelled me to forsake a rather mediocre tennis game for fun on the paddle tennis court. There, thanks to much-maligned lobs and drop and cut shots, a tennis player lives again.

—Robert Andresen

As George Burns often said, "You can't avoid growing older, but you don't have to get old." A person must stay active mentally and physically.

—Bill Witter

Growing older is easy. You just continue to have birthdays. There are advantages. Not much is expected of you in your eighties. So you relax and actually play a better game, and it's more fun. I play better paddle tennis now than I did at seventy-two. And my golf game is getting steadier.

—John Siemens

Close friends and hearty companions, members of the coed Villa Marin Paddle Tennis Team meet twice each week to do battle with racquets and balls. They enjoy the camaraderie and teasing as much as the exercise, which keeps them youthful and vital.

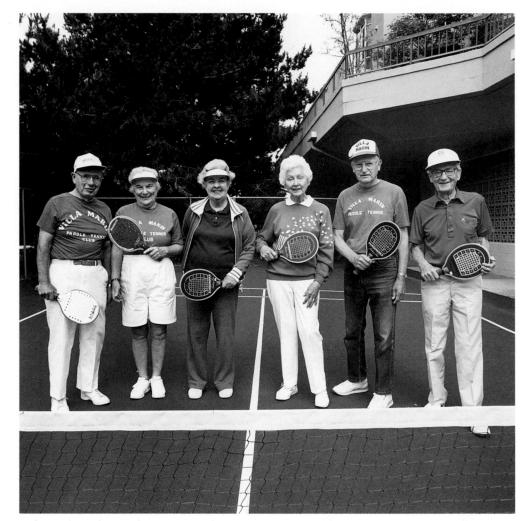

Left to right: Robert Andresen, Roma Bloom, Jane Bennett, Dodie Greve, John Siemens, Bill Witter

E. MURIEL BENNETT

Paddle tennis player, age 83

Years of age make for nervousness and assume importance only on the application for a driver's license renewal. Otherwise, fame comes from mental or physical exploits. Paddle tennis is my game.

—*E. Muriel Bennett*

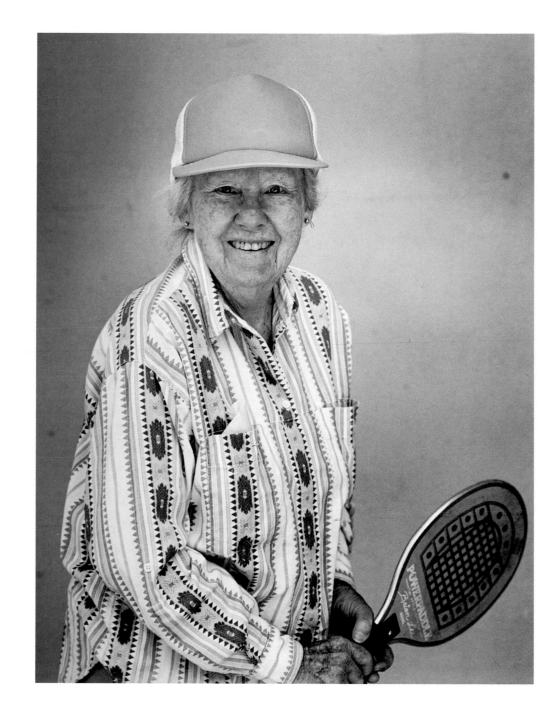

NORMA TEAGARDEN-FRIEDLANDER

Jazz pianist, age 84

I've been very lucky to love what I do and have the good health to do it. Also, I've been blessed with so many good friends and to have been a member of a talented and loving family. I seldom meet a person I don't like.

—*Norma Teagarden-Friedlander*

A member of the famous Teagarden jazz family (her brothers, Jack, Charlie, and Cub, were all jazz greats during the 1930s, 1940s, and 1950s), Norma is a San Francisco legend in her own right. She is the city's "Grand Lady of Jazz" and knocks 'em out nightly on piano at various clubs and joints, getting a good workout in the process. She also entertains regularly at local convalescent hospitals.

Members of her jazz group are, from left, Fred Anderson (clarinet), Waldo Carter (trumpet), and Brian Richardson (trombone); not shown is Don Bennett (bass).

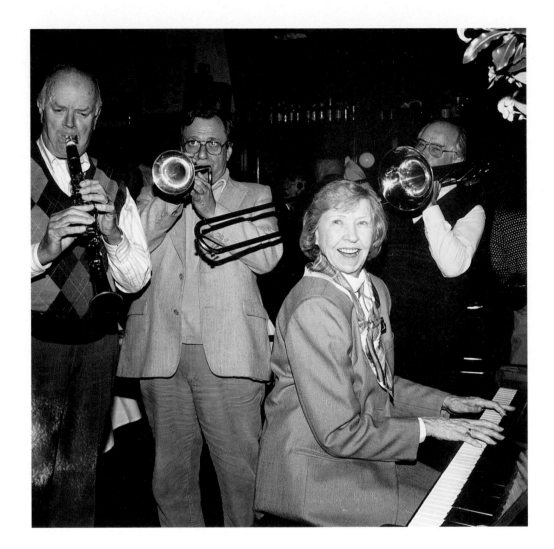

ANNA HALPRIN

Dancer, age 75

Dance has been an inspiration and joy throughout my whole life. It has been a way for me to live my life fully, and it has healed me. Dance is my favorite way of being with others and sharing my vision of a creative and peaceful world.

—*Anna Halprin*

Anna founded the San Francisco Dancers' Workshop forty years ago. In 1978 she started the Tamalpa Institute in Marin County, California, where she teaches dance as a healing aid and as a performing art. Anna survived cancer and believes she was cured by dancing. Among her many achievements and awards are a Guggenheim Fellowship, the American Dance Guild award for outstanding contributions in the field of dance, and the Sustained Achievement award from the Bay Area Isadora Duncan Hall of Fame.

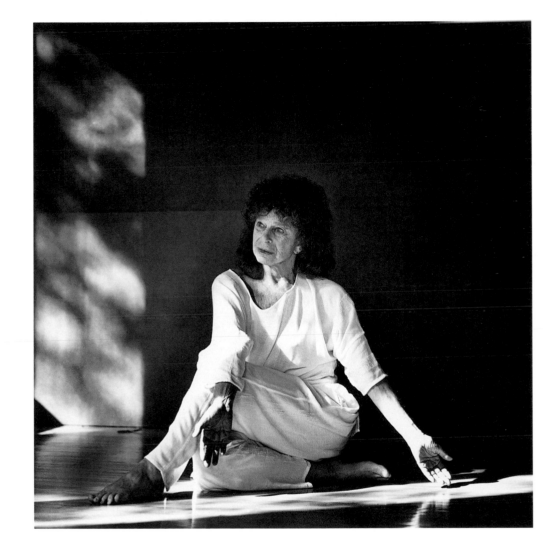

SUN CITY
AQUA SUNS

Synchronized swimmers, ages 68–88

Synchronized swimming is sometimes called "dancing underwater." The Aqua Suns practice their complex synchronized patterns for many hours to achieve near perfection and compete at the national level in the Senior Olympics. Like Esther Williams, they perform with ease, grace, and always a smile!

Opposite page, left to right: Georgia Clark, Peggy Kaems, Hope Hathaway, Helen Edwards, Iris Mitrick, Pat Johnson

Page 70, left to right: Grace Jurincic, Betty Coffey, Gertrude Flesh, Shirley Muise, Mary Pat Wagner, Lorraine Carriyeau (also pictured on this page and page 71 with two other members of their group who I couldn't catch in time to photograph)

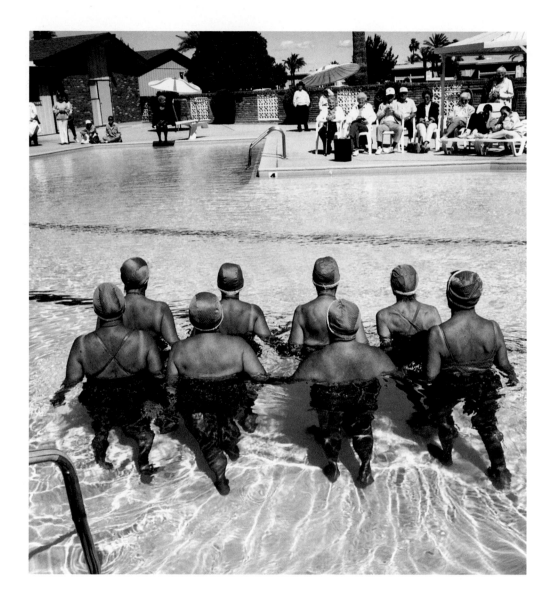

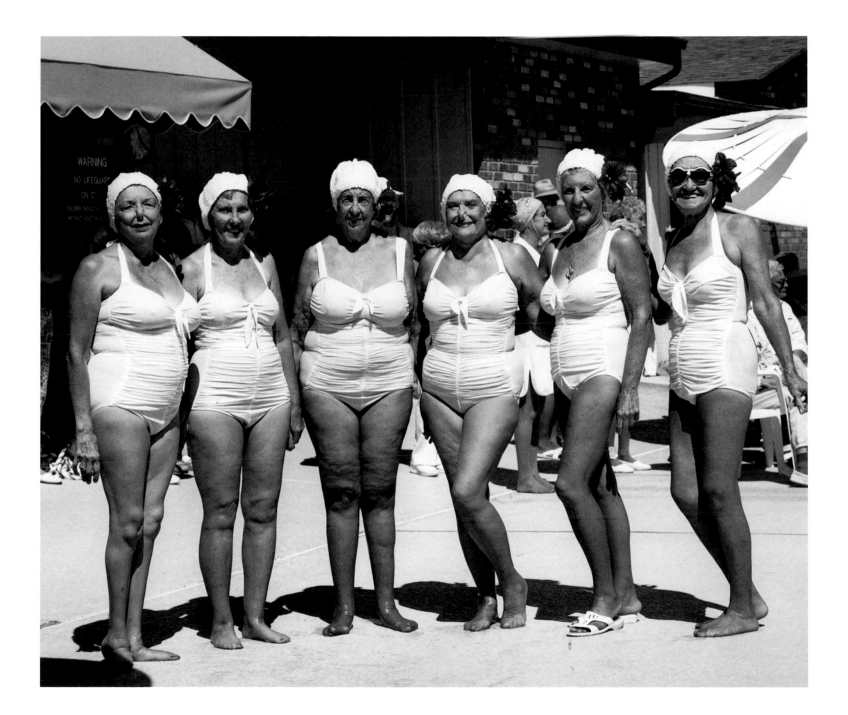

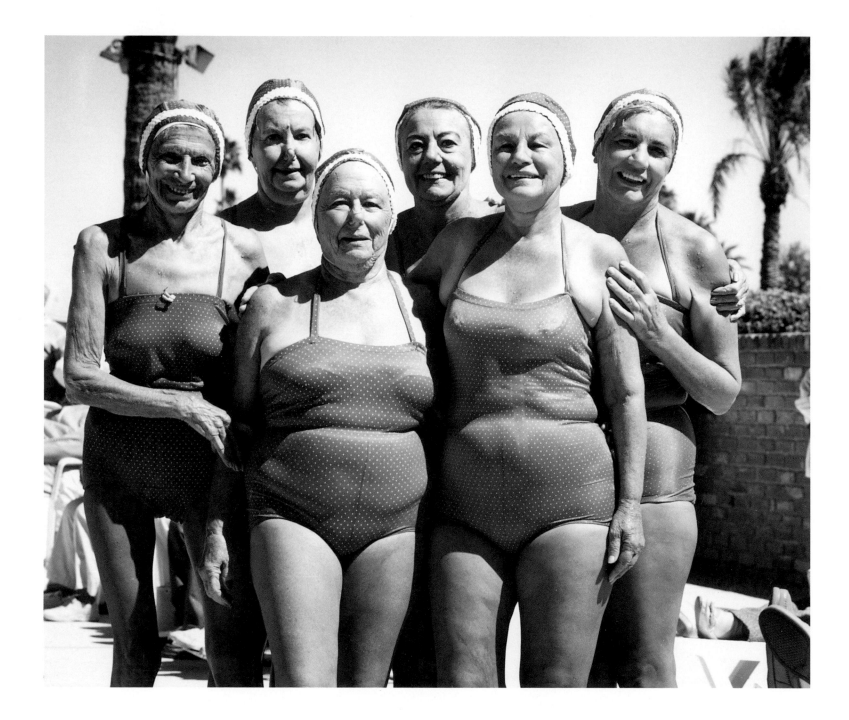

70

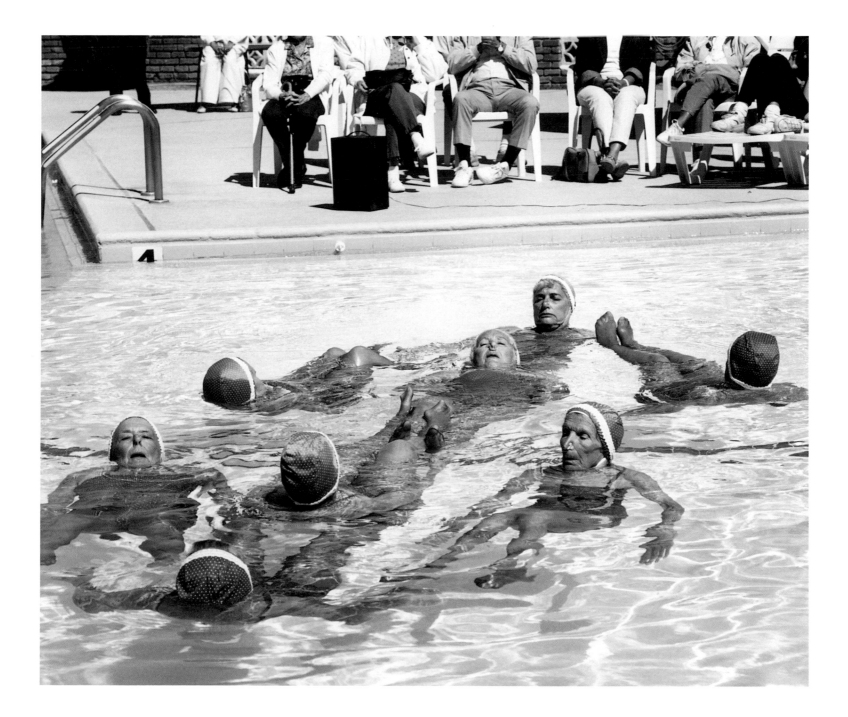

INGEBORG NATOLI
AND MARY McBAIN

Synchronized swimmers, ages 65
and mid-70s, respectively

Synchronized swimming is the passion that drives Mary's and Ingeborg's lives. They work out six days a week, for three to five hours a day, and compete in national and international meets whenever they can. Mary's latest accomplishment is winning a gold medal in the sixty to sixty-nine age group for her exquisite solo performance in the 1994 Senior National Championships in Scottsdale, Arizona. She is currently in training for next year's games. Ingeborg won a gold medal in her age category in the same competition and plans to repeat her achievement next year.

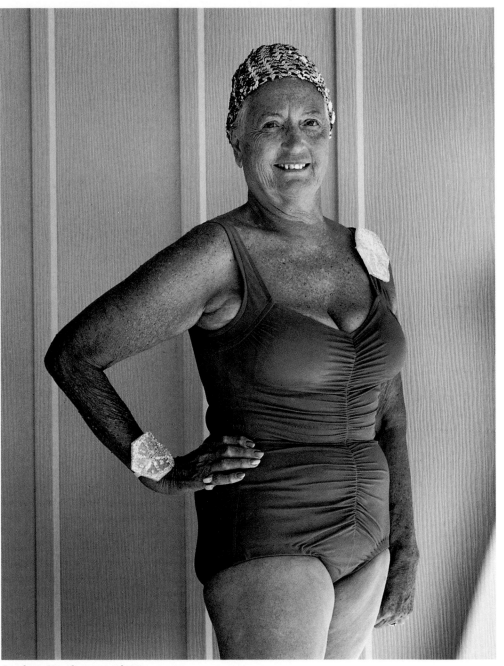

Ingeborg Natoli, age mid-70s

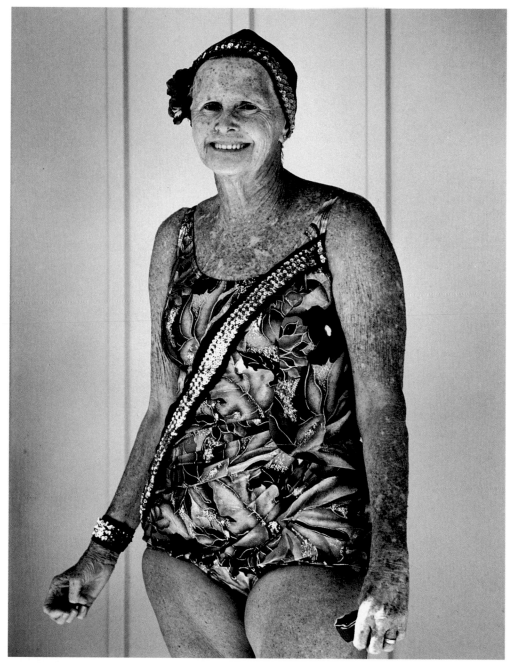

Mary McBain, age 65

CLIFF "ANGEL" FARFEL

Skier, age 74

Known as the guardian angel of the Purgatory, Colorado, ski area, Cliff skis the slopes, checking skiers' equipment for potential safety hazards and helping people in trouble. He got his nickname years ago when he rescued a man and his daughter who were lost on the snowy mountain. They were both suffering from hypothermia, the girl worse than the father. Cliff helped them off the mountain and left without giving them his name. The man called the Purgatory Ski Patrol and described the mystery savior as an angel. The name stuck.

Cliff loves his job on the mountain. "I grew up once, and I didn't like it. I didn't have anyone to play with," he says. Now he plays all day in the snow.

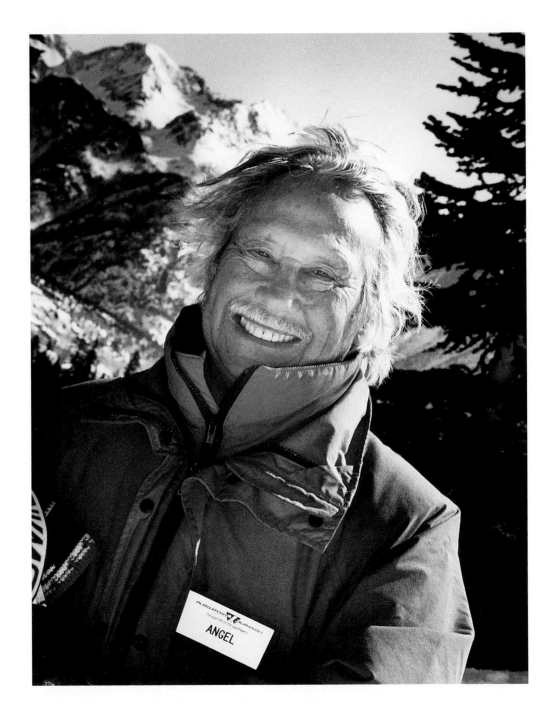

MARIAN (HAAS) ANDERSON

Skier, age 74

I do not wear a watch or keep a calendar, remembering my current age with some difficulty. Each day to me is a new adventure, unrelated to what has gone before or what will follow. I am optimistic about my capabilities and intolerant of the limitations my bones would impose. I love babies and require the presence of children and young adults in my life. Variety is also important—the change of scenes and seasons. Life, for the most part, has been very good to me, and if I had it to do over again, I would do it entirely differently—just for fun!

—*Marian Anderson*

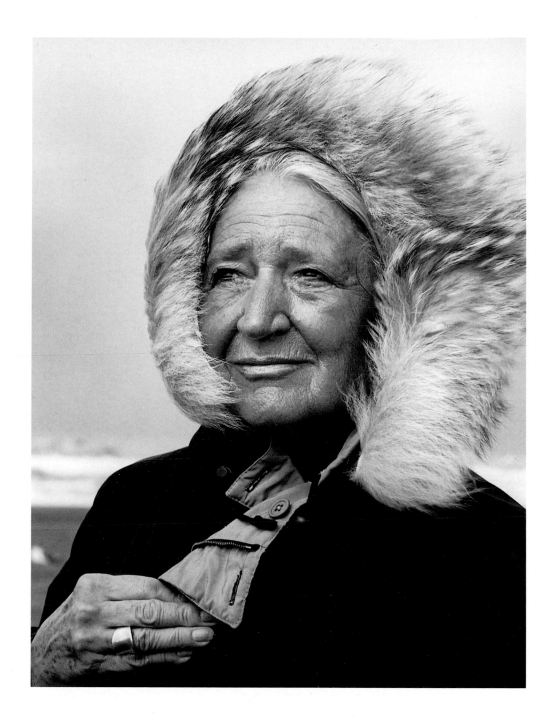

ALAN BENEFIEL, ROBERT JACOBSON, BOB BEERS, AND CLIFF "ANGEL" FARFEL

Skiers, ages 61, 71, 80, and 74, respectively

These four skiers rule the Purgatory, Colorado, ski area. Robert and Bob are employed as certified ski instructors, and Alan and Angel are mountain "binding mechanics" who act as angels for those who have broken bindings or limbs.

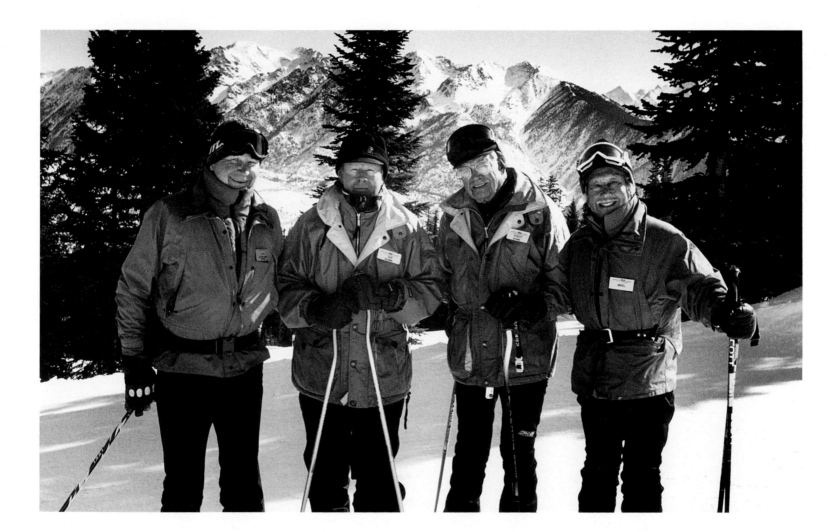

BOB BEERS

Skier, age 80

"Old skiers never die; they just slide down-hill," says Bob Beers, who has been a passion-ate skier for four decades.

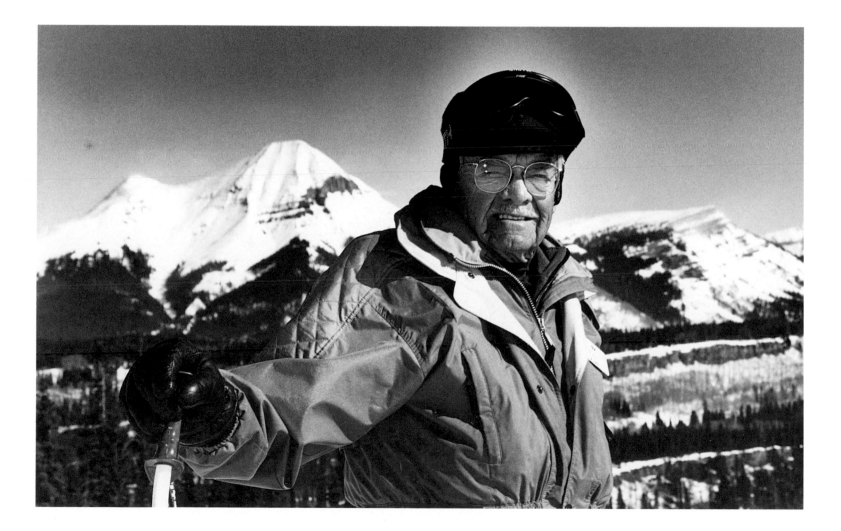

CARL YATES

Ultra marathoner, age 68

Don't give up. If you don't use it, you lose it.

—*Carl Yates*

Carl has completed nine 100-mile runs, including the country's four most difficult 100-mile trail runs, the Hardrock 100, the Wasatch, the Superior, and the Angeles Crest. He also competes in fifty-kilometer ski races and snowshoe marathons. His training schedule before a race includes two days of long workouts (twelve to fifteen hours) and three to five short days of a mere four to six hours.

Carl told me about a strange incident he experienced during one of his runs. "I was doing a relatively easy 100-mile race in Arkansas and was about 75 miles into it. I fell asleep running. I woke up in time to keep going—but started running in the wrong direction."

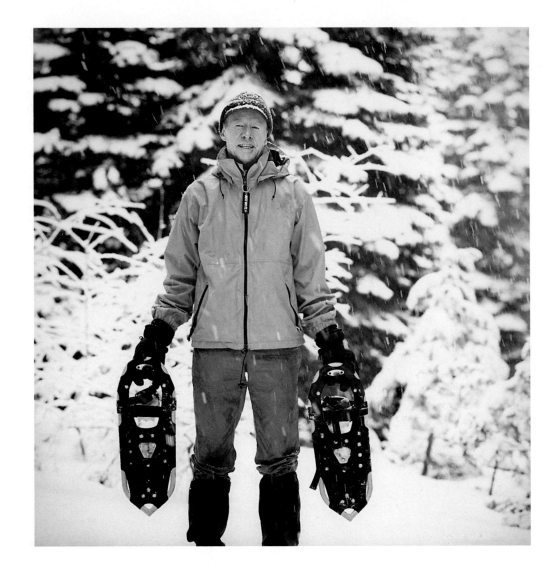

ROY ERLANDSON

Swimmer, age 82

Roy began his competitive swimming career as a sixty-year-old rookie looking for a form of exercise under doctor's orders. He had developed asthma and emphysema and needed to turn his life around. "If I didn't swim, I would be dead by now," he says. He loves the swim meets because he "meets very nice people." Here are Roy's rules of life.

Take time to think—
    it is the source of power.
Take time to play—
    it is the secret of perpetual youth.
Take time to read—
    it is the fountain of wisdom.
Take time to pray—
    it is the greatest power on earth.
Take time to love and be loved—
    it is a God-given privilege.
Take time to be friendly—
    it is the road to happiness.
Take time to laugh—
    it is the music of the soul.
Take time to give—
    it is too short a day to be selfish.
Take time to have faith—
    it is the key to Heaven.

—Roy Erlandson

GOLFERS

Average age 75

*These golfers from Sun City, Arizona, rang-
ing in age from seventy to eighty, are among
the best players on the Arizona seniors circuit.
Most of them picked up the sport late in life.
A few have scores lower than their ages, and
the rest are trying.*

*Front row, left to right: Rosemary Schultz,
Mary Wold, June Sitts, Leone Grandy, Dottie
Stewart*

*Back row, left to right: Betty Welch, Sandy
Wadas, Myrtle Siegel*

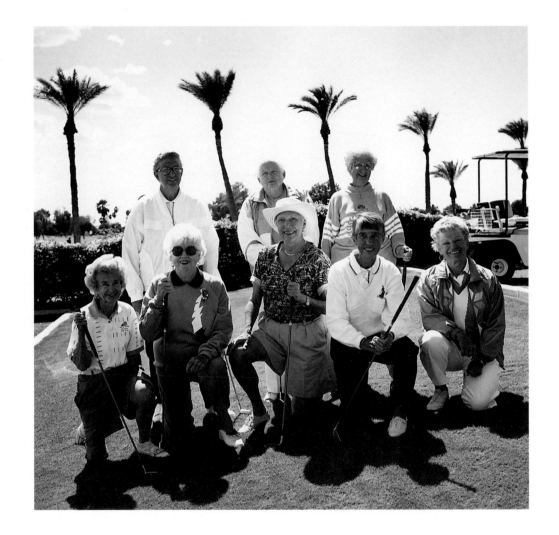

ROSEMARY SCHULTZ

Golfer, age 81

At age seventy-nine, Rosemary was nearly crippled with rheumatoid arthritis—enough, one might think, to end the career of any golfer. But not Rosemary's! She was determined to keep playing, and with the help of physical therapy she made a remarkable comeback on the links, where she still plays every day.

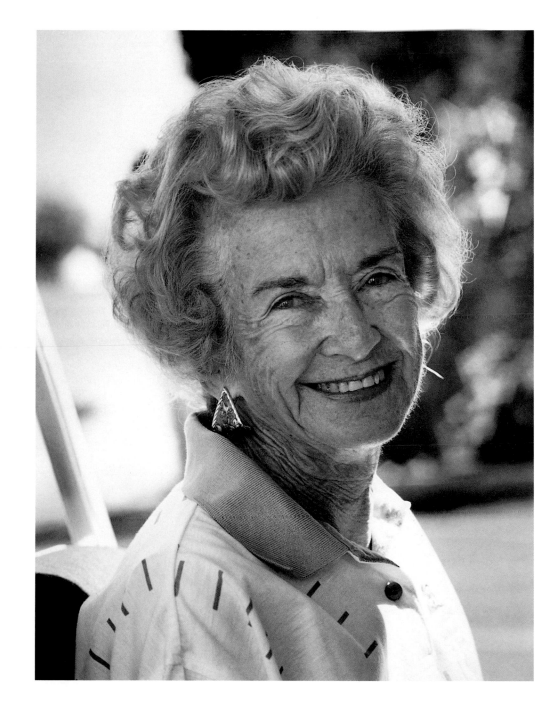

WAIKIKI OPEN-WATER SWIM

About two thousand hardy open-water swimmers plunge into the breaking surf of Waikiki Beach at the start of the 1994 race. Not everyone finished the grueling 2.7-mile course, which was punctuated by strong currents, head winds, and dangerous riptides. But everyone survived.

Most of the swimmers I photographed for this book have competed at least once in the annual Waikiki Open. It seems to be a rite of passage for long-distance swimmers of all ages.

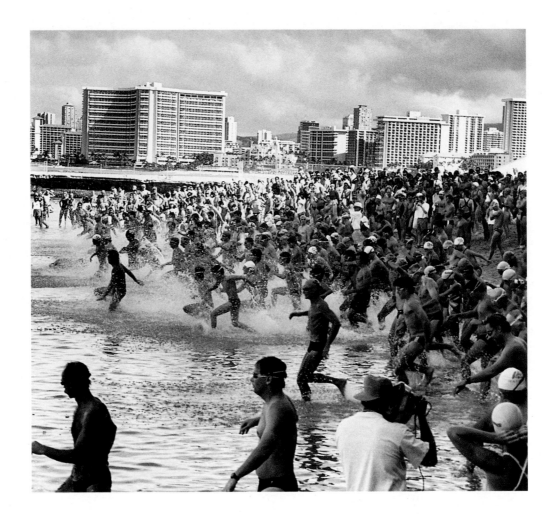

ZADA AND RAY TAFT

Swimmers, age 76

We were lucky to develop a common interest in the sport and spent weekends body surfing and surfboarding. We liked the workouts, our teammates, and good, clean, healthy living. True, true, we lose some of our physical strength and concentration in our present life, but with what we have left, there is no better way to activate our endorphins than swimming and competing.

—*Zada and Ray Taft*

Known as the "king and queen of masters swimming," Zada and Ray have been swimming together since they first met in the water in 1936. Zada has swum San Francisco's Golden Gate twenty-two times, has competed in the annual race around Alcatraz Island a dozen times, and is currently a member of two national record-setting relay teams. Ray holds eight world masters short course records in freestyle swimming. He also holds several world and national records in the long course. Ray has competed in twenty of the challenging annual Waikiki Open-Water Swims. The latest was in 1994.

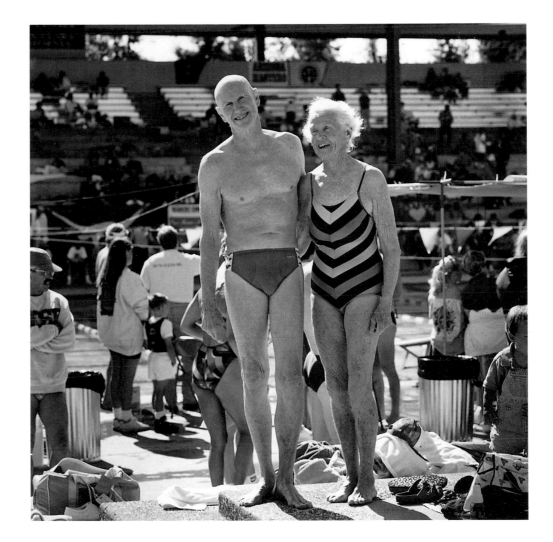

MASTERS
SWIMMERS

Average age: 71

These four gents are members of the San Francisco Olympic Club's masters relay team. They consistently take medals in national meets, but they enjoy the camaraderie as much as the competition. When I called Ed Rudloff, he explained the team's casual philosophy: "We're not very good swimmers and have never scored in first place as a relay team, but individually we have done quite well."

Left to right: Ralph Perry, Glynn Jones, Frank Grannis, Ed Rudloff

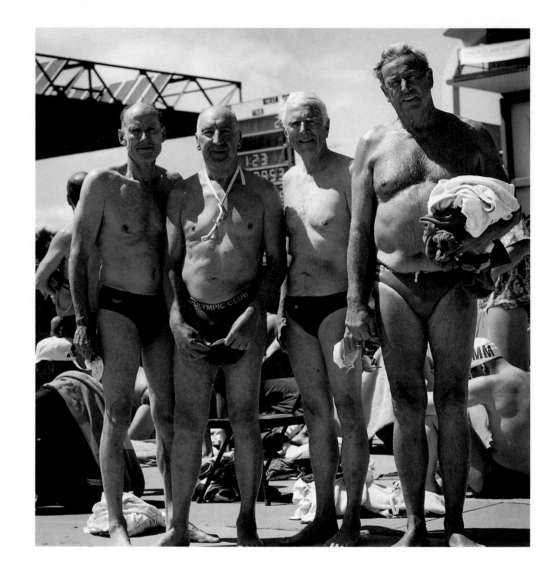

WINNING RELAY SWIM TEAM MEMBERS

These four swimmers, pictured here at the Santa Clara national swim meet, had just won the gold medals in the individual medley relay and the freestyle relay. This meant they were the best in the United States in their age bracket, seventy-five to eighty.

Left to right:

Mary Jane Reeves, age 78
"I show up at the pool four to five times a week and do as I am told. I eat whatever I want and stop when I am full."

Frieda Sidorsky, age 79
Frieda's training methods are: swim five days a week from 5:30 A.M. to 6:45 A.M. She eats everything.

Jean Durston, age 81
Jean swims four days a week and eats everything.

Sally Joy, age 78
"My philosophy of life is 'Do the best you can with what you have been given.' Strive to overcome adversity and be happy. Either you overcome a handicap or you are overcome by it."

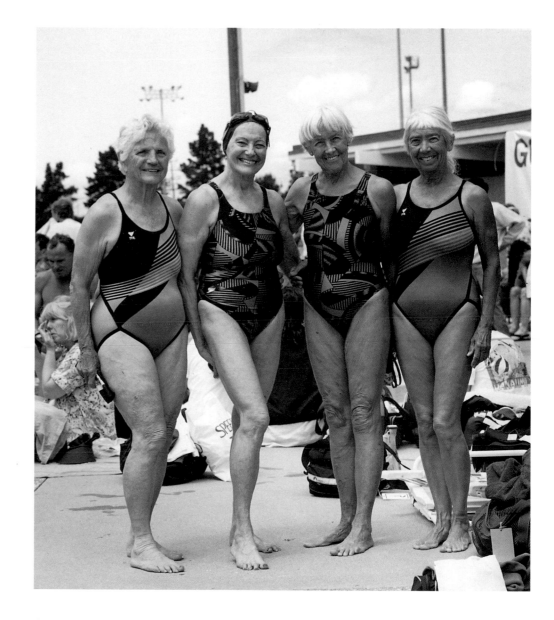

GERRY WILSON

Exerciser, age 60

Gerry, a graphic designer who has a pet llama, is a former runner. His knees gave out a few years ago, forcing him to create his own workout regimen. His ten-minute workout, which he has found to be a youthful elixir, includes stretching, 200 abdominal crunches, 100 push-ups, and "roll-outs" on his exercise wheel. This short but vigorous routine keeps him at a trim and muscular 160 pounds— only five pounds more than he weighed in high school, when he was a three-sport athlete.

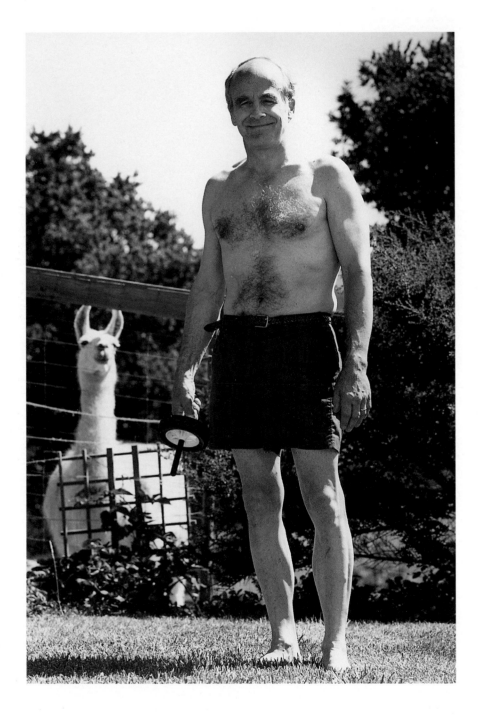

DWIGHT STRONG
AND
JENNINGS SMITH

Fencers, ages 79 and 78, respectively

Dwight (left) and Jennings (right) are both former college fencers who took up the sport again later in life. Nearly half a century after graduation, Dwight, a painter and collector of African art, resumed fencing at the age of sixty-nine to get into shape for backpacking and mountain climbing. He got into great shape and has been fencing ever since. Jennings, treasurer of the U.S. Olympic Fencing Association, returned to fencing at age forty-nine, following back surgery, and has taken on all comers of any age or gender with the saber. He also competes in national masters tournaments.

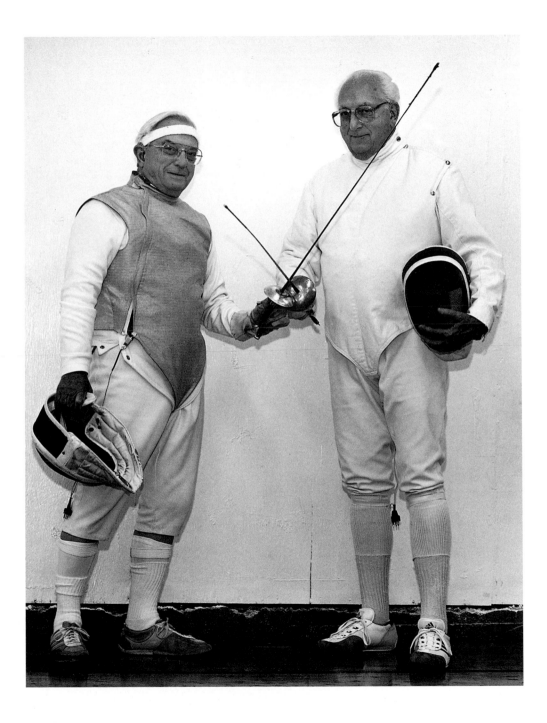

LOIS ANDERSON

Tai chi and kung fu student, age 68

I was a dance teacher for most of my life and began to realize that I could transform my body's attributes and condition by the way I directed it with my mind. I didn't realize I had a mind-body connection at work, since at the time no one talked about it that way.

I smoked cigarettes for thirty-seven years but quit eleven years ago. I replaced the habit immediately with Chinese herbs and active, steady tai chi and kung fu programs. I was determined to construct a healthy survival program of my own making. Martial arts have given me stamina, health, strength, and a lifelong commitment to rejuvenation.

—*Lois Anderson*

Lois is both a martial arts student and a sensuous dancer and performance artist.

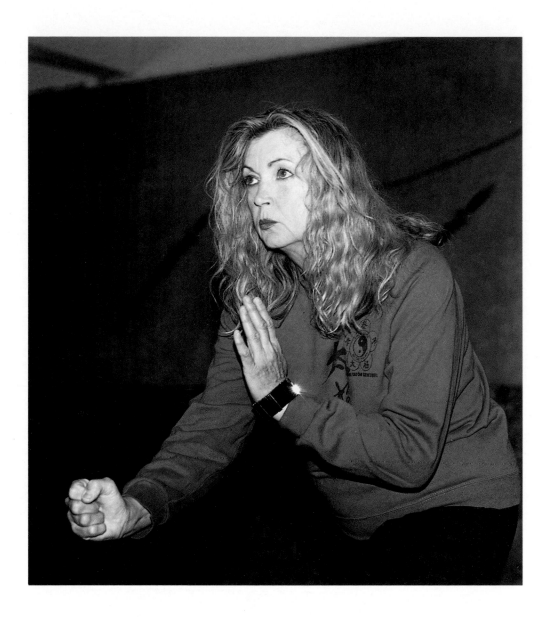

ED BRUNETTI

Weight lifter, age 70

Ed is a retired butcher who has worked out and lifted weights since he was a boy. The results of his lifelong zeal are evident in his bulging forearms and rippling abs. His training advice: "Just start in and do it. But start real slow."

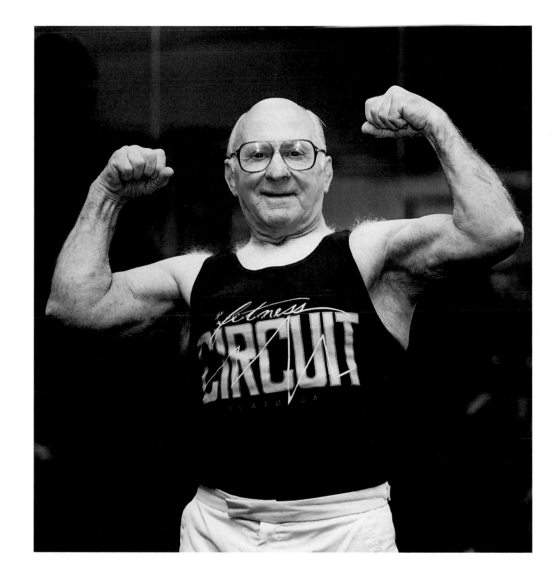

ADELINE "TIGER" SHRAPNEL

Surfer, age 75

Adeline, known as "Tiger" on Waikiki Beach, had a radical mastectomy in 1975. Two years later she had a second mastectomy. "Surfing kept me going and made life worth living," says Tiger, who surfs every day except Sundays. "There is always another wave."

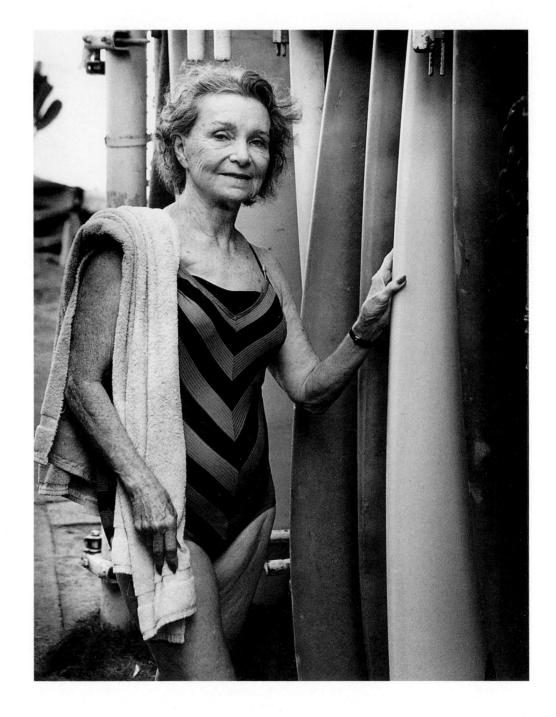

EDWARD B. RANDOLPH

Surfer, age 73

I am too immature to have developed a philosophy of life, but I like the following, which I read somewhere eons ago: "Nothing matters; everything counts."

—*Edward B. Randolph*

When I asked Edward to tell me his major athletic accomplishments, he replied, "Learning to surf at age forty-seven." His training methods include meditation before surfing. He quit smoking twenty-five years ago. He eats only when hungry and drinks wine but no hard liquor. His dislikes: "The manners, music, and lack of intellectual development of the past three generations. And anybody as intolerant as I am!" His loves: "Ladies; dogs; people who are articulate and kind; young children; all gentle earthlings, human or otherwise."

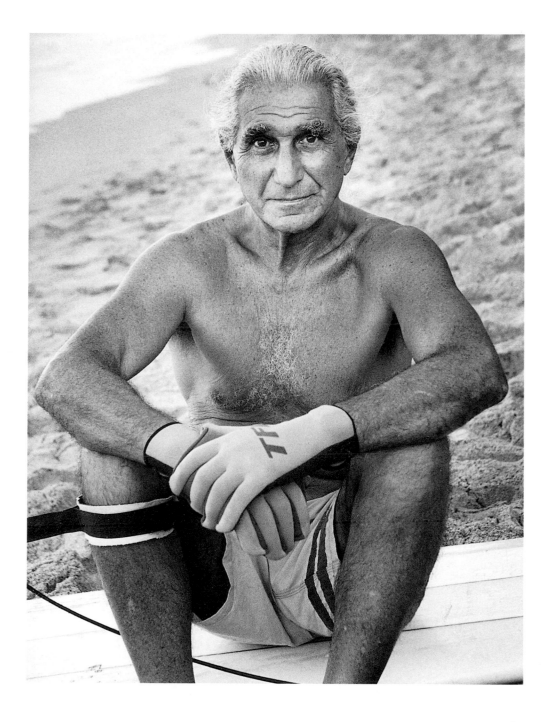

MARIN ROWING ASSOCIATION MEMBERS

Average age: 76

These eight rowers meet at least twice a week to row and train for masters eight-man crew races around the country. They have won numerous championships, despite shoulder and hip replacements and several coronary bypasses.

Back row, left to right: Jerome Lerner, John Adams, Bert Danziger, Roger Barbie, Roger Thompson, Bill Tuinzing, Cam Jones, Carleton Whitehead

Front row, left to right: Burton Ballard, coxswain; Tim Ryan, coach

Believe me, my young friend, there is nothing—absolutely nothing—half so much worth doing as simply messing about in boats.

—*from* The Wind in the Willows
by Kenneth Grahame

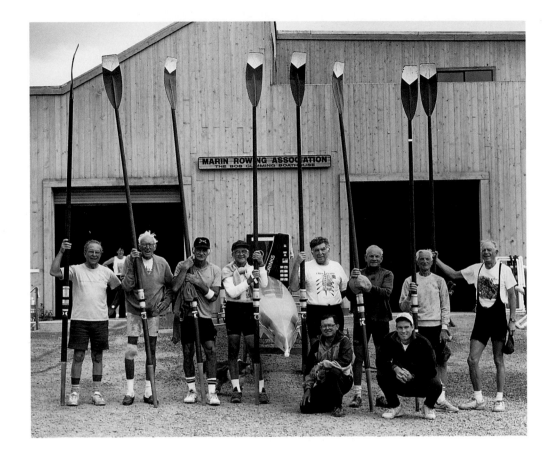

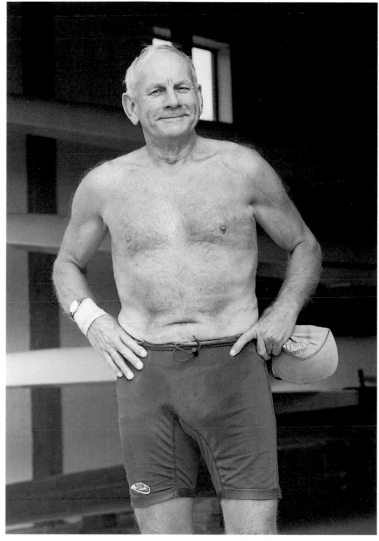

Bill Tuinzing

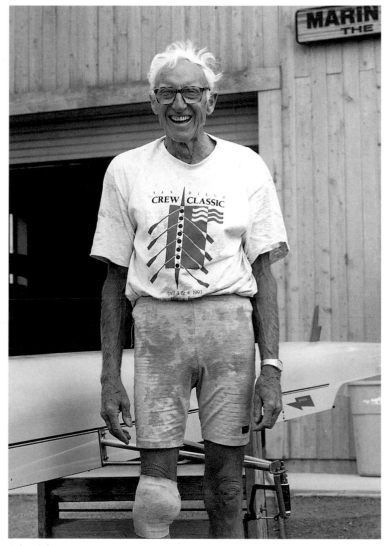

John Adams

LANDON CARTER

Rower, age 52

Rowing is a sensual sport. As the boat goes through the water, you can feel the water move underneath you. You can hear the boat move—a sensual sound—a kind of swish as it cuts through the water.

—*Landon Carter*

Landon, the youngest athlete in this book, started rowing when he was forty-eight. Two years later, he became the U.S. National Masters Single Scull champion. He served as the rabbit that the older rowers tried to catch.

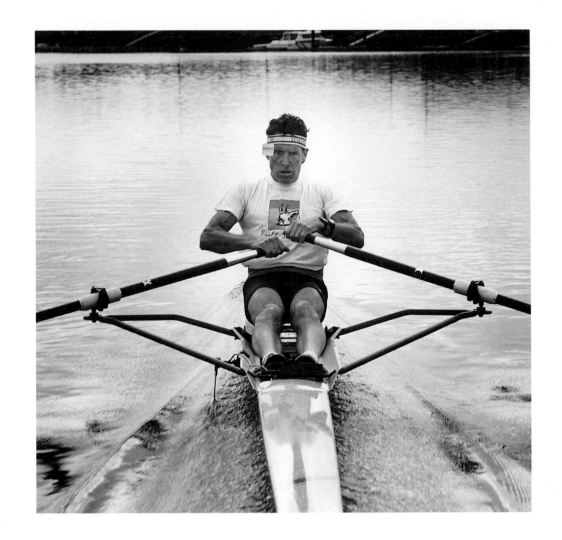

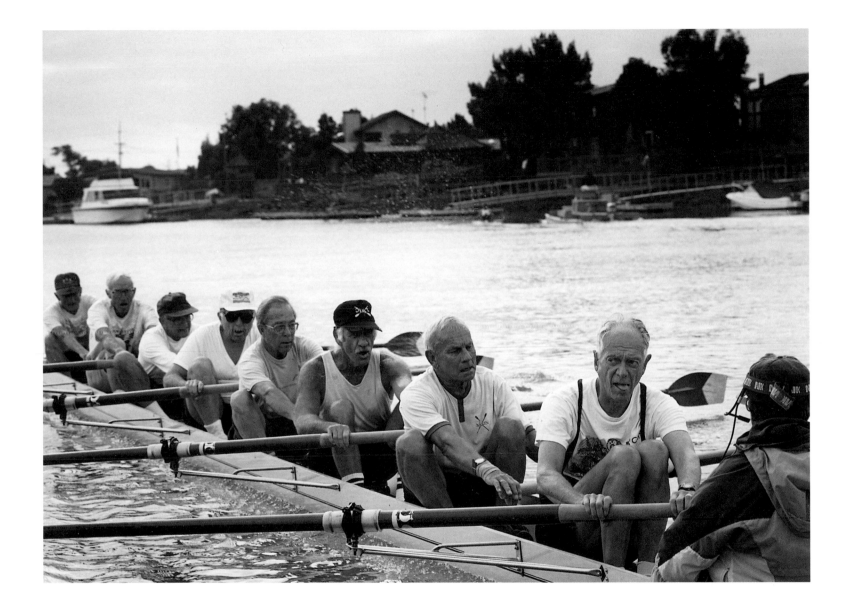

DONALD GOO

Surfer, age 73

"Just live and don't let yourself get old," says
Donald *("Mr. Magoo" to his buddies), who
surfs the heavies of his native Hawaii.*

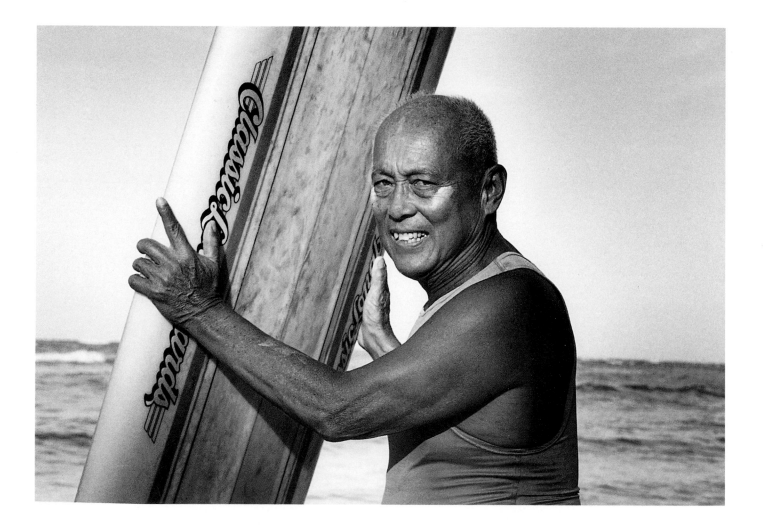

MILDRED BALL-WILSON

Surfer, age 75

In 1989, one year after my first husband passed away, I met Harry Ball-Wilson of London, England. He had been guided to Hawaii by his late wife, through a spirit medium, to find me. The spirit said I would be a perfect partner for him. We were married in London, and together we believe that it is love that makes the world go 'round.

—*Mildred Ball-Wilson*

Mildred is a familiar figure on the Waikiki strip. Not only does she surf every day, but often she can be seen kayaking along the shore.

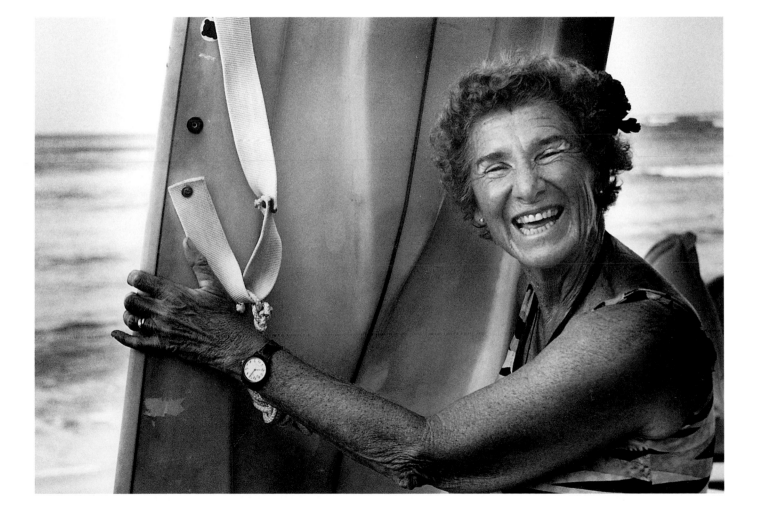

ALBERT J. MARENHOLZ

Polo player, age 75

Albert and his horse, Classy Stuff, have competed in hundreds of polo matches over the years. He keeps and trains three horses in order to compete with the youngsters, since "there aren't many old guys like me riding polo."

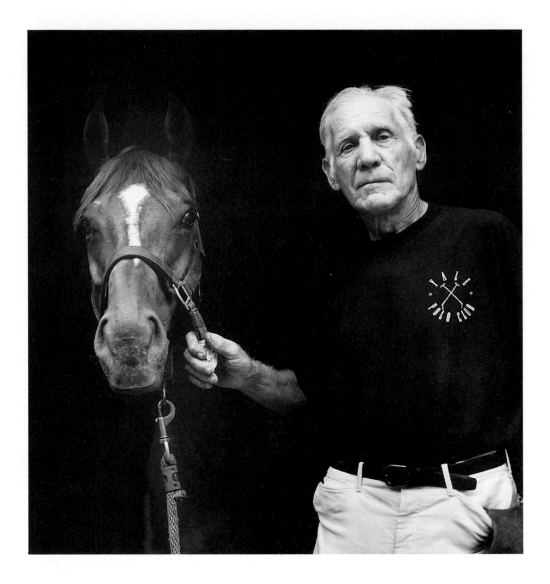

OSBORN "OZZIE" HOWES

Horse trainer and rider, age 72

I've never accomplished anything except reaching seventy-two by a fairly comfortable route. I have been physically active by default, there being little intellectual competition. Reading is swell for an hour or two, but then I just have to bust loose and do something. I like to smoke a pipe after dinner and enjoy a couple of bourbon or gin cocktails before. Plenty of red meat. Big bacon-and-egg breakfasts four times a week, with cereal or pancakes alternatively.

—*Ozzie Howes*

I photographed Ozzie resting in the sun while he was helping train and break some horses that had been brought to the Humane Society, where he volunteers his services.

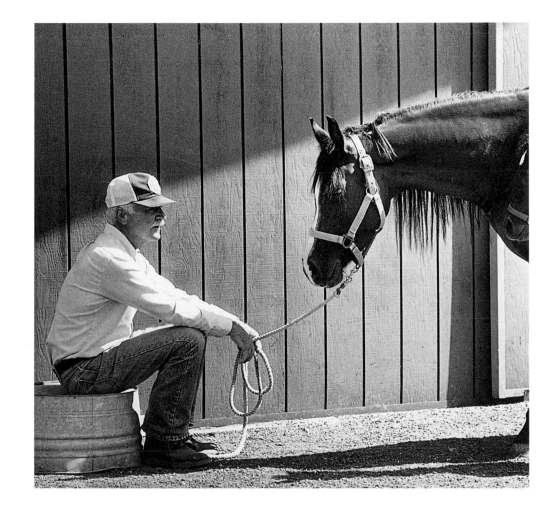

ANNA AND TONI WILLINGER

Hikers, age 68

I met Anna and Toni on a bus trip through the Southwest. They had come from Austria to visit and hike the national parks. Anna told me that she'd had a stroke and her doctor had told her she would never be able to climb mountains and hike again. With the help of her husband, Toni, she recovered, and they celebrated the miracle with a tour of the United States. When I first saw Anna she was standing high up on a ledge in Arches National Park, Utah, giving her husband a big kiss.

To me, fair friend,
You can never be old.
For as you were
When first your eye I eyed,
Such seems your beauty still.

—*William Shakespeare*

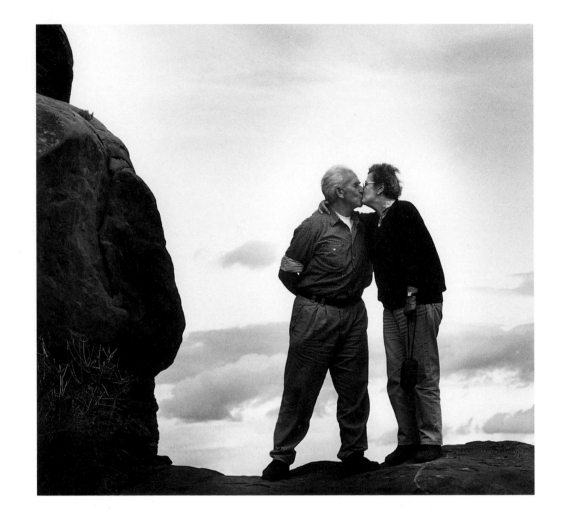

JIM AND ELAINE GREENLEE

Bungee jumpers, age 68

Typical "snowbirds" who ply our highways and byways during the year, Jim and Elaine follow the seasons in their very plush 1935 GMC 4104 bus. I caught up with them in Durango, Colorado, where they were flying glider planes. They spend many hours at various fairs looking for excitement, and they are accomplished bungee jumpers. Next, they would like to try hot air ballooning. Their philosophy: "Live the best you can today, and be kind and friendly. Tomorrow will take care of itself."

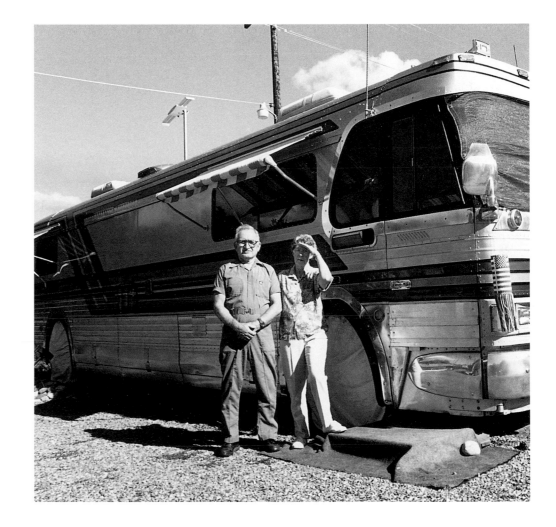

OLA EIKREM

Mountain climber and bird counter, age 74

Ola is the second woman to have climbed every one of the fifty-four peaks over 14,000 feet high between Canada and Mexico. She still hikes and climbs, but I caught up with her at one of her more relaxing activities, counting migrating birds, at Stinson Beach, north of San Francisco. Her husband, Bjorn, claims Ola is the strongest female hiker in California. "What other woman has climbed all of the 14,000-foot peaks, and what other woman can hike fifty-five miles and climb 15,000 feet with a heavy load in three days?" he boasts.

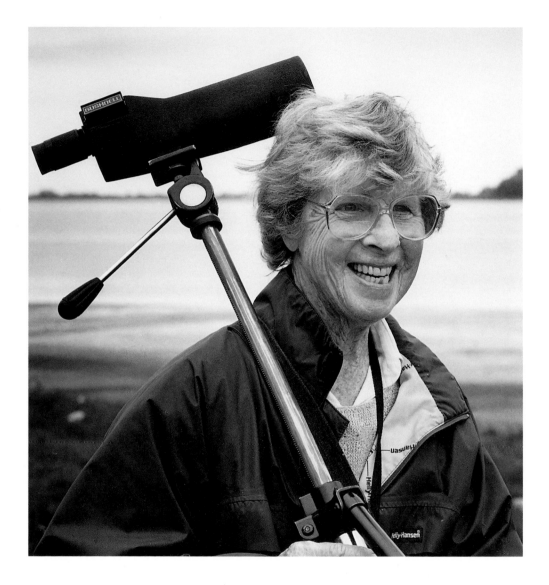

BJORN EIKREM

Hiker and mountain climber, age 80

Here is an old Norse tale Bjorn told me. Thor was known as the mightiest of the Norse gods. Once, when in the land of the giants, he challenged the giants to a wrestling match. But none of them would accept the challenge, so their chief called an old woman, who agreed to the wrestling match. After a violent struggle, she succeeded in bringing Thor down to one knee, and the giants called a stop to the match. Later, the chief of the giants told Thor that he had done remarkably well, as he was actually wrestling with Old Age, and there never was, and never will be, a man whom Old Age will not sooner or later lay low.

"If, as this story tells us, old age and its consequences are inevitable to those lucky enough," Bjorn concludes, "one had best find ways to enjoy old age while it lasts."

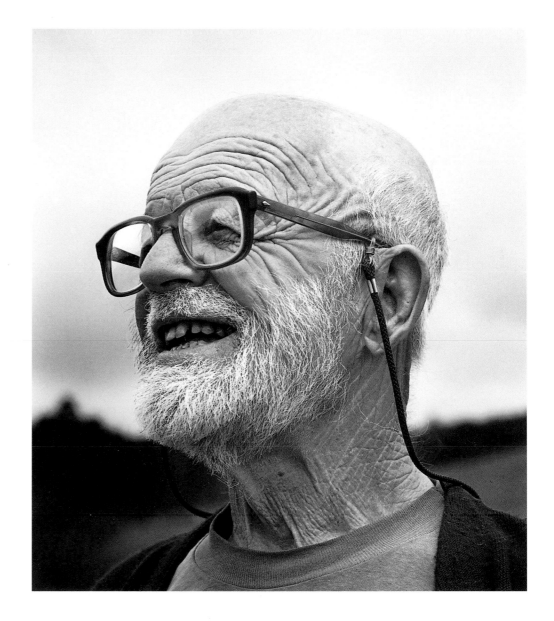

"COWBOY" ROSA

Surfer, age 58

Known as "the mayor of Waikiki," Cowboy is a fixture on Waikiki Beach. He is easy to pick out of a crowd with his giant twelve-and-a-half-foot surfboard, which he claims is the biggest in Hawaii. A native of Honolulu, Cowboy has been a master surfer since his teen years, when he took on the challenging and treacherous Haleiwa Pipeline and Sunset at the age of fifteen. He has taught surfing on Waikiki Beach for the past twenty years. Besides being a surfer, Cowboy is a big game hunter, an accomplished skin diver, and a master chef.

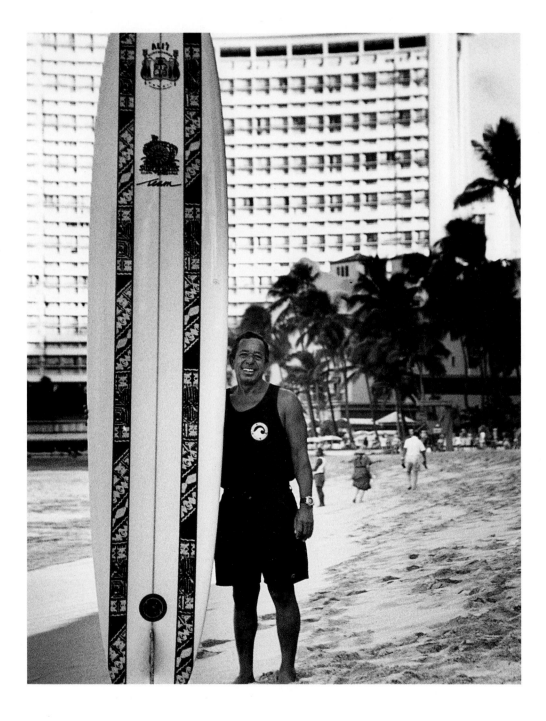

RUSS QUAINTANCE

Surfer, age 80

Russ was an accomplished surfer long before the sport became popular on the U.S. main-land. He started in 1932 with the heavy boards, then polished his skills during World War II in the surf of Iwo Jima, where he and his buddies built their own boards out of material that had been damaged in battle and discarded. Now, in gentler surroundings, Russ surfs and socializes every day at sunrise on Waikiki Beach.

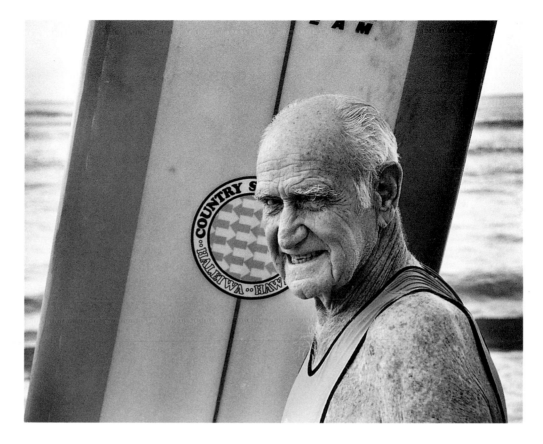

WALTER POMORIN
AND
HANS LUCHTERHAND

Runners, mid-60s

Walter (left) and Hans (right) are avid long-distance runners from Villingen, Germany, whose ambition has always been to run across San Francisco's famous Golden Gate Bridge. They finally fulfilled their dream during a recent California vacation. I caught them under the North Tower of the bridge just as they were finishing their run.

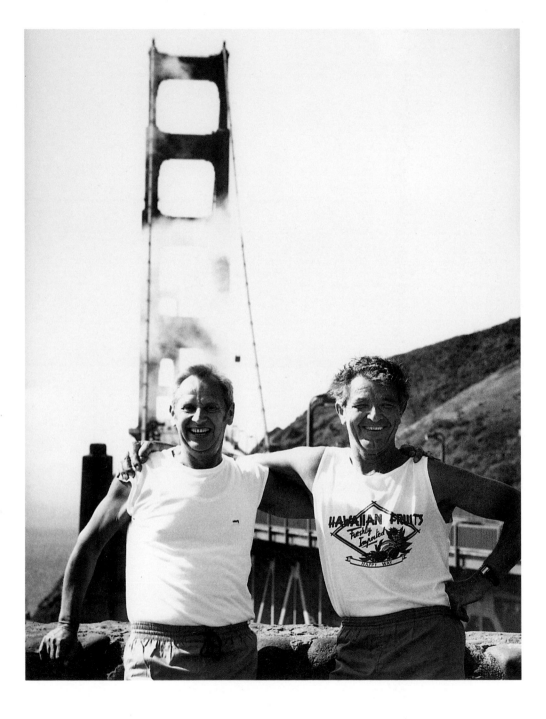

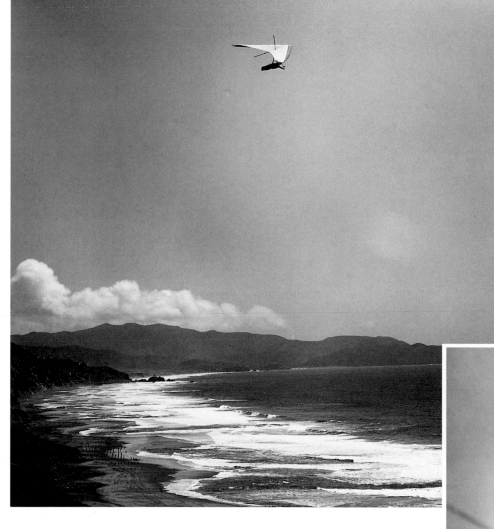

ROBERT BYRD

Hang glider, age 74

Life is short, so enjoy every minute. Hang gliding, for me, lifts the spirits and recharges the old batteries. It is the greatest sport going, and lots of exercise too.

—*Robert Byrd*

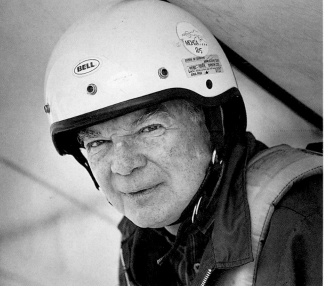

IDA KLINE

Aerobics instructor, age 100

The secret to staying young at heart is staying fit; the key to a long life is to control your worries. I don't worry about tomorrow. If you have a problem and you can't fix it, you should dismiss it from your mind. So many people waste time worrying when they could be thinking pleasant thoughts.

The best part of living is the people in the world; there are so many wonderful people. That's what keeps me going.

—*Ida Kline*

Ida teaches aerobics and stretching every day and practices yoga.

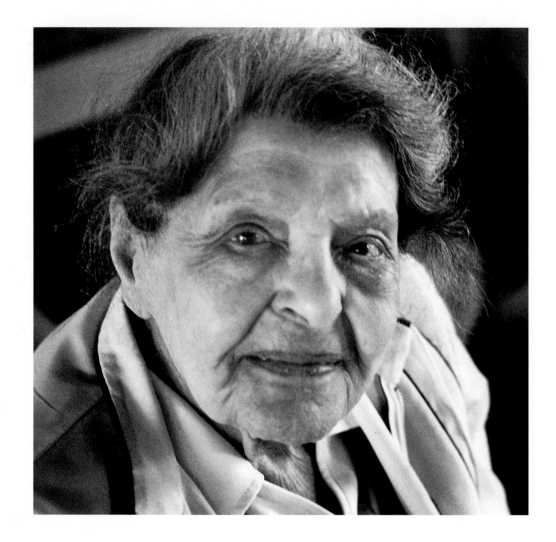

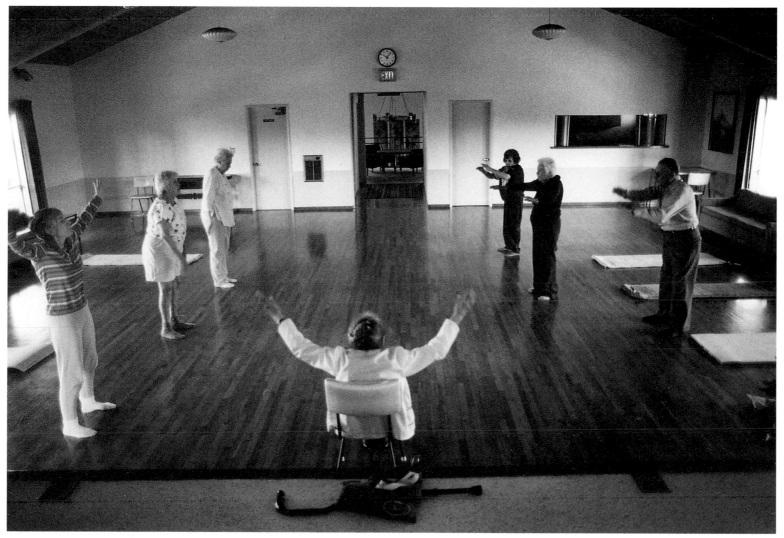

Ida Kline, age 100, with her aerobics and stretching class

JOE VARRELLI

Line, round, and square dancer, age 70

Joe is a popular figure in Arizona's country dancing community. He specializes in square, round, and line dancing, as a dancer, caller, and teacher. When he is not on the road calling square dances around the country, Joe teaches about 650 students a week in Sun City.

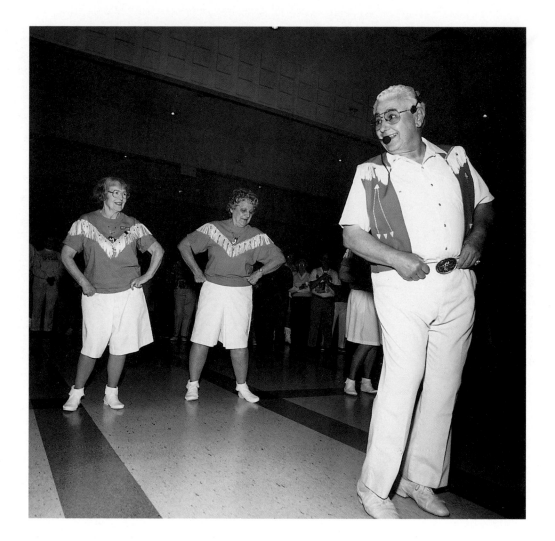

LILO STOJANOVIC
AND PAUL SCHMIDT

Dancers, ages mid-70s and 90, respectively

Paul and Lilo were cutting a mean rug at Ritter's Dance Club in Sun City, Arizona, when I caught up with them for this shot. They didn't say much except that they love to dance together, and then they spun away.

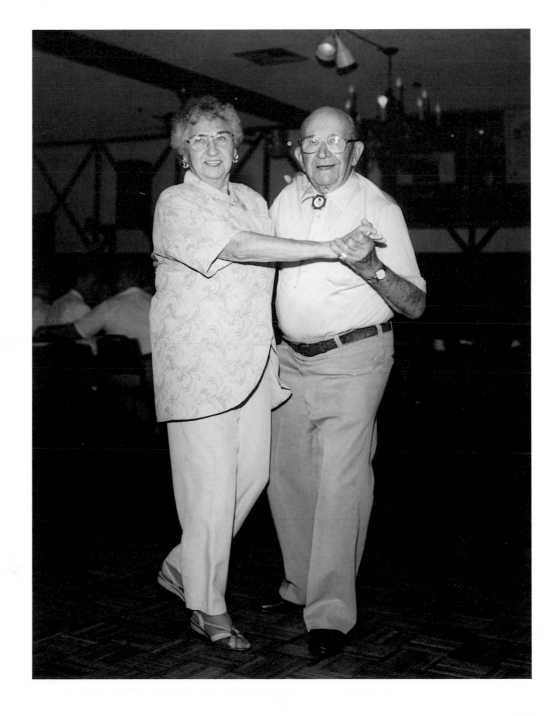

ED LONGNER

Bowler, age 93

When Ed was ninety, he bowled a 611 series to clinch the eighty-plus handicap play at the 1992 Valleywide Senior Bowling Event in Scottsdale, Arizona. He was the oldest competitor and topped nineteen bowlers in the eighty-and-over competition. He also won a bronze medal in bowling at the 1988 Arizona Senior Olympics.

Ed believes he is able to participate in sports at his age because of a moderate exercise regimen and a vegetarian diet. He did not start bowling until he was seventy-four. He stands on his head five minutes every day and calls it "reverse aging."

Ed's business card reads:

no phone   no address

Retired

"When I have the urge to work, I lie down until the urge passes."

no business   no money

no prospects   no worries

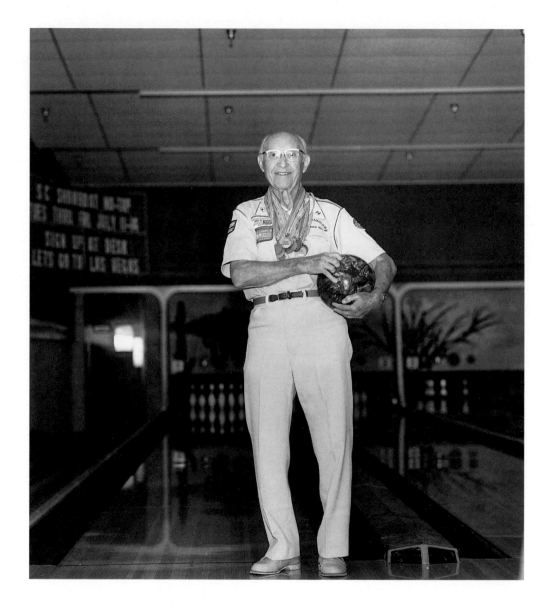

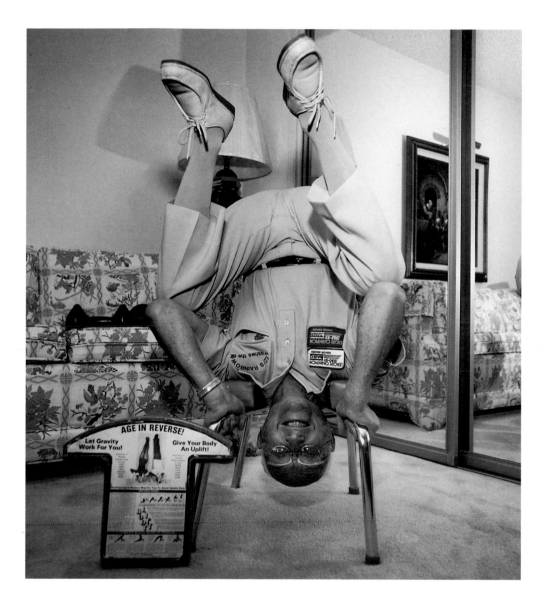